From Neurobiology to Treatment:

Bipolar Disorder and Schizophrenia Unraveled

Every effort has been made in preparing this book to provide accurate and up-to-date information that is in accord with accepted standards and practice at the time of publication. Nevertheless, the author, editors, and publisher can make no warranties that the information contained herein is totally free from error, not least because clinical standards are constantly changing through research and regulation. The author, editors, and publisher therefore disclaim all liability for direct or consequential damages resulting from the use of material contained in this book. Readers are strongly advised to pay careful attention to information provided by the manufacturer of any drugs or equipment that they plan to use.

PUBLISHED BY NEI PRESS, an imprint of NEUROSCIENCE EDUCATION INSTITUTE
Carlsbad, California, United States of America

NEUROSCIENCE EDUCATION INSTITUTE
1930 Palomar Point Way, Suite 101
Carlsbad, California 92008

http://www.neiglobal.com

Printed in the United States of America
First Edition, August 2009

Typeset in Myriad Pro

Library of Congress Cataloging-in-Publication Data
ISBN 1-4225-0051-9

Table of Contents

CME Information

Overview
The successful treatment of bipolar disorders and schizophrenia depends largely on a proper diagnosis and on adherence to pharmacotherapy. This booklet will unravel the neurobiology underlying these two disorders and will explain the mechanisms of action of medications used to treat both disorders. Individual medications will be discussed as well as switching strategies.

Target Audience
This CME activity has been developed for MDs specializing in psychiatry. There are no prerequisites for this activity. Physicians in all specialties who are interested in psychopharmacology, as well as nurses, psychologists, and pharmacists, are welcome for advanced study.

Statement of Need
The following unmet needs regarding bipolar disorder and schizophrenia were revealed following a critical analysis of activity feedback, expert faculty assessment, literature review, and through new medical knowledge:

- Acute treatments for bipolar disorder often result in syndromal remission but rarely in full functional remission; this is at least partially due to the inadequacy of maintenance therapies currently available.
- Different classes of mood stabilizers have different pharmacological properties leading to different efficacies and side effects depending on a myriad of variables.
- Although many clinicians generalize that higher doses are associated with greater efficacy and more side effects, the efficacy and tolerability profile for different doses of some mood stabilizers are far less straightforward than that.
- Schizophrenia is one of the most debilitating psychological disorders associated with the worst quality-of-life and lowest remission rates.
- Patients respond to atypical antipsychotics in individual and often unpredictable ways. A cache of side effects is associated with treatments for psychosis, including uncomfortable adverse reactions and risk of serious health problems, both of which can lead to problems with patient adherence.
- Some newer treatments for schizophrenia are turning out to have different optimum dosing techniques and broader clinical applications than expected.

To help fill these unmet needs, quality improvement efforts need to:

1) Improve understanding of the neurobiology of bipolar disorders and the pharmacology of available, new, and in-development medications
2) Improve understanding of the neurobiology of schizophrenia and the pharmacology of available, new, and in-development medications

Learning Objectives
After completing this activity, participants should be better able to fulfill the following learning objectives:

- Describe the hypothetical neurobiology of bipolar disorders and the complex pharmacology of mood stabilizers used to treat them
- Recognize how different drugs affect the various disease states of bipolar disorders and identify mechanisms as well as therapeutic benefits and nuances of drugs commonly prescribed for bipolar disorder
- Develop an understanding of the best treatment practices and maintenance methods for optimizing individual patient outcome in bipolar disorder
- Describe the hypothetical neurobiology of schizophrenia and understand the complex pharmacology of antipsychotics
- Recognize how different drug properties affect the various symptoms of schizophrenia and that side effects are linked to the drug's receptor profile
- Develop an understanding of the best treatment practices and switching methods in schizophrenia

Accreditation and Credit Designation Statements

The Neuroscience Education Institute is accredited by the Accreditation Council for Continuing Medical Education to provide continuing medical education for physicians.

The Neuroscience Education Institute designates this educational activity for a maximum of 3.0 *AMA PRA Category 1 Credits*™. Physicians should only claim credit commensurate with the extent of their participation in the activity. Also available will be a certificate of participation for completing this activity.

Nurses in most states may claim full credit for activities approved for *AMA PRA Category 1 Credits*™ (for up to half of their recertification credit requirements). This activity is designated for 3.0 *AMA PRA Category 1 Credits*™.

Activity Instructions

This CME activity is in the form of a printed monograph and incorporates instructional design to enhance your retention of the information and pharmacological concepts that are being presented. You are advised to go through the figures in this activity from beginning to end, followed by the text, and then complete the posttest and activity evaluation. The estimated time for completion of this activity is 3.0 hours.

Instructions for CME Credit

To receive your certificate of CME credit or participation, please complete the posttest (you must score at least 70% to receive credit) and activity evaluation found at the end of the monograph and mail or fax them to the address/number provided. Once received, your posttest will be graded and a certificate sent if a score of 70% or more was attained. Alternatively, **you may complete the posttest and activity evaluation online and immediately print your certificate**. There is no fee for CME credits for this activity.

NEI Disclosure Policy

It is the policy of the Neuroscience Education Institute to ensure balance, independence, objectivity, and scientific rigor in all its educational activities. Therefore, all individuals in a position to influence or control content development are required by NEI to disclose any financial relationships or apparent conflicts of interest that may have a direct bearing on the subject matter of the activity. Although potential conflicts of interest are identified and resolved prior to the activity being presented, it remains for the participant to determine whether outside interests reflect a possible bias in either the exposition or the conclusions presented.

These materials have been peer-reviewed to ensure the scientific accuracy and medical relevance of information presented and its independence from commercial bias. The Neuroscience Education Institute takes responsibility for the content, quality, and scientific integrity of this CME activity.

Individual Disclosure Statements
Author
Laurence Mignon, PhD
Senior Medical Writer, Neuroscience Education Institute, Carlsbad, CA
Stockholder: Aspreva Pharmaceuticals Corporation; Vanda Pharmaceuticals Inc.; ViroPharma Incorporated

Content Editors
Meghan Grady
Director, Content Development, Neuroscience Education Institute, Carlsbad, CA
No other financial relationships to disclose.

Stephen M. Stahl, MD, PhD
Adjunct Professor, Department of Psychiatry, University of California, San Diego School of Medicine, San Diego, CA
Grant/Research: Forest; Johnson & Johnson; Novartis; Organon; Pamlab; Pfizer; Sepracor; Shire; Takeda; Vanda; Wyeth
Consultant/Advisor: Arena; Azur; Bionevia; Boehringer Ingelheim; Bristol-Myers Squibb; CeNeRx; Dainippon Sumitomo; Eli Lilly; Endo; Forest; Janssen; Jazz; Johnson & Johnson; Labopharm; Lundbeck; Marinus; Neuronetics; Novartis; Noven; Pamlab; Pfizer; Pierre Fabre; Sanofi-Synthélabo; Sepracor; Servier; Shire; SK; Solvay; Somaxon; Tetragenix; Vanda
Speakers Bureau: Pfizer; Wyeth

Peer Reviewer
Ronnie Gorman Swift, MD
Professor and Associate Chairman, Department of Psychiatry and Behavioral Sciences, New York Medical College, Valhalla, NY; Professor of Clinical Public Health, School of Public Health New York, New York Medical College, Valhalla, NY; Chief of Psychiatry and Associate Medical Director, Metropolitan Hospital Center, New York, NY
No other financial relationships to disclose.

Design Staff
Nancy Muntner
Director, Medical Illustrations, Neuroscience Education Institute, Carlsbad, CA
No other financial relationships to disclose.

Disclosed financial relationships have been reviewed by the Neuroscience Education Institute CME Advisory Board to resolve any potential conflicts of interest. All faculty and planning committee members have attested that their financial relationships do not affect their ability to present well-balanced, evidence-based content for this activity.

Disclosure of Off-Label Use
This educational activity may include discussion of products or devices that are not currently labeled for such use by the FDA. Please consult the product prescribing information for full disclosure of labeled uses.

Disclaimer
The information presented in this educational activity is not meant to define a standard of care, nor is it intended to dictate an exclusive course of patient management. Any procedures, medications, or other courses of diagnosis or treatment discussed or suggested in this educational activity should not be used by clinicians without full evaluation of their patients' conditions and possible contraindications or dangers in use, review of any applicable manufacturer's product information, and comparison with recommendations of other authorities. Primary references and full prescribing information should be consulted.

Participants have an implied responsibility to use the newly acquired information from this activity to enhance patient outcomes and their own professional development. The participant should use his/her clinical judgment, knowledge, experience, and diagnostic decision-making before applying any information, whether provided here or by others, for any professional use.

Grant Information
This activity is supported by educational grants from Bristol-Myers Squibb Company and Lilly USA, LLC. For further information concerning Lilly grant funding visit, www.lillygrantoffice.com.

Chapter 1

Spectrum of Bipolar Disorders: From Symptoms to Circuits to Neurotransmitters and Mechanisms

Chapter 1 aims to describe the hypothetical neurobiology of bipolar disorders. This chapter introduces the symptoms of bipolar disorders from depression to mania. Patients with bipolar depression often present with nearly identical symptoms as patients with unipolar depression, and recognizing differences between these disorders can therefore be difficult. Patients with bipolar disorder often seek help during periods of depression and report manic symptoms with less frequency, further complicating diagnosis. Although bipolar II disorder is increasingly diagnosed, it is still quite often overlooked or misdiagnosed as unipolar depression, anxiety, or other psychiatric illnesses.

Understanding the neurobiological nature of an illness is the first step in deciding how to treat it. Identifying circuits that hypothetically correspond to the major symptoms of mania and depression becomes especially critical when attempting to establish pharmacologic parallels to treat those symptoms. Although much is still unknown about the aberrant circuitry in bipolar disorder, the brain regions and circuits that are theoretically involved are under intense investigation.

Mood Chart

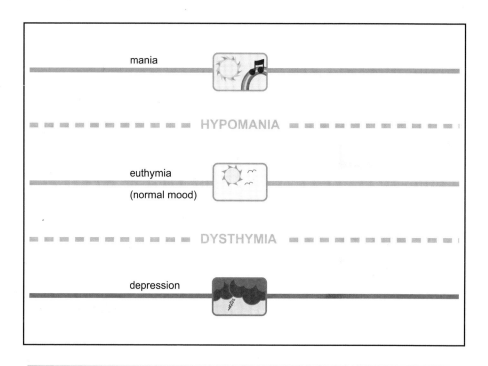

FIGURE 1.1. Mood charts illustrate a spectrum of normal and pathological states upon which a patient's mood can be charted over time. Mood monitoring can be conducted intermittently in a clinical setting or continuously via patient self-report in the form of a mood diary. Bipolar patients present a particularly difficult diagnostic challenge, as this disorder often manifests in complex moods that can change over time. Tracking the course of illness can greatly assist in identifying disease states, diagnosing accurately, and assessing treatment response. This chart illustrates definitions of disease states: hypomania is a less severe, shorter-lasting form of mania, and dysthymia is a less severe, longer-lasting form of depression.

What Proportion of Mood Disorders Are Bipolar?

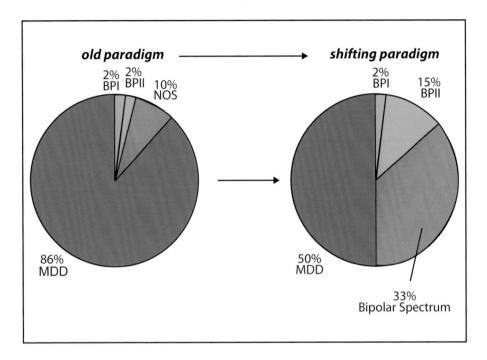

FIGURE 1.2. Diagnoses of bipolar disorder have become increasingly common in recent years. Although many patients who would have previously been diagnosed with major depressive disorder are now being diagnosed with bipolar disorder, the syndrome can be hard to detect. There is still a large proportion of patients who go many years without an accurate diagnosis of bipolar disorder; the most common mis-diagnosis is overwhelmingly major depressive disorder, followed by anxiety disorder, schizophrenia, and borderline/antisocial personality disorders.

Identifying Mood Disorders:
Bipolar I vs. Bipolar II

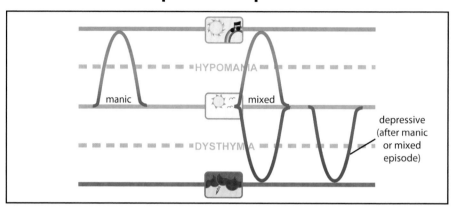

FIGURE 1.3. A mood chart for bipolar I disorder is characterized by manic or mixed episodes, with or without major depressive episodes. Patients with bipolar I disorder spend more time in the manic or hypomanic phase as compared to patients with bipolar II disorder. Patients with bipolar I disorder also exhibit higher rates of reckless activity, distractibility, agitated activity, irritable mood, and increased self-esteem as compared to patients with bipolar II disorder.

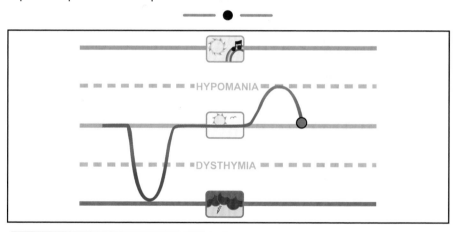

FIGURE 1.4. A mood chart for bipolar II disorder is characterized by major depressive and hypomanic episode(s). Patients with bipolar II disorder spend more time in the depressed phase and less time asymptomatic compared to patients with bipolar I disorder. Patients with bipolar II disorder also exhibit a higher lifetime prevalence of shorter inter-episode intervals, more rapid onset, and more comorbid anxiety disorders as compared to patients with bipolar I disorder.

Symptoms of Depression and Mania

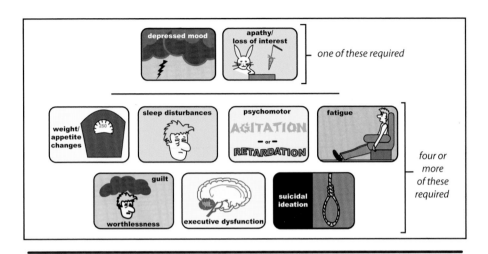

FIGURE 1.5. These are the symptoms of depression as designated by the Diagnostic and Statistical Manual of Mental Disorders, fourth edition (DSM-IV). According to these criteria, diagnosis of a major depressive episode requires at least one of the symptoms in the top row as well as at least four of the symptoms in the bottom two rows.

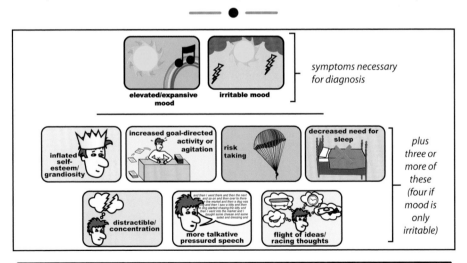

FIGURE 1.6. These are the symptoms of mania as designated by the DSM-IV. According to these criteria, diagnosis of a manic episode requires at least one of the symptoms in the top row as well as at least three of the symptoms in the bottom two rows. Four of the symptoms in the bottom two rows are required if the mood is only irritable.

Unipolar vs. Bipolar Depression?
Check the History

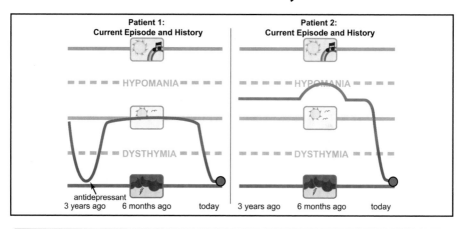

FIGURE 1.7. Although both patients in this mood chart are "today" presenting with identical current symptoms of a major depressive episode, patient 1 has unipolar depression while patient 2 has bipolar depression. So, what is the difference? The pattern of past symptoms is quite different and relevant, with patient 1 having experienced a prior depressive episode and patient 2 a prior hypomanic episode. Gaining a complete picture may often require additional interviews with family members or close friends of the patient.

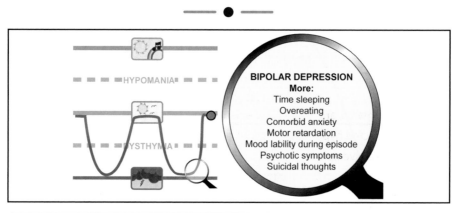

FIGURE 1.8. Although they can occur in either disorder, some symptoms of depression are more prevalent or frequent in bipolar depression than in unipolar depression. Observing patients' sleep and eating habits and looking for the presence of anxiety, motor slowing, mood lability, psychotic symptoms, and/or suicidal ideation can aid in differentiating bipolar from unipolar depression.

The Bipolar Spectrum

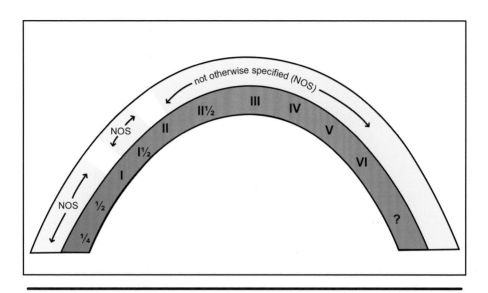

FIGURE 1.9. The DSM-IV distinguishes only between bipolar (I and II), and cyclothymic disorder, classifying all presentations that do not fit these categories as "not otherwise specified (NOS)." This might be conceptually inadequate due to the dramatic variation in presentation within the NOS category. It may be more accurate to conceptualize all bipolar disorders on a spectrum such as the one simplified here.

"Not Otherwise Specified" Bipolar Disorders	
¼	Depressive episodes but rapid poop-out to antidepressants
½	Schizobipolar disorder: Positive symptoms of psychosis with manic, hypomanic, and depressive episodes
I ½	Protracted hypomania without depression
II ½	Depressive episodes with cyclothymic temperament
III	Depressive episodes with antidepressant-induced hypomania
III ½	Bipolar disorder, substance abuse
IV	Depressive episodes with hyperthymic temperament
V	Depression with mixed hypomania
VI	Bipolarity in the setting of dementia

TABLE 1.1. Characterization of "NOS" bipolar disorders.

Circuits in Depression

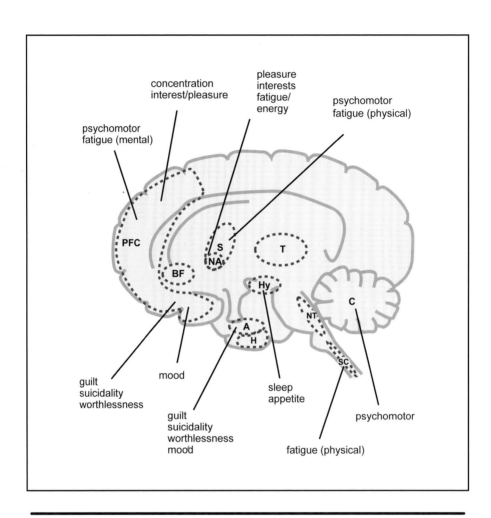

FIGURE 1.10. Various brain regions are hypothetically associated with particular symptoms of depression, and aberrant neuronal activity in any of these brain regions can theoretically lead to symptoms of a major depressive episode. The following several pages examine each of these symptoms and regions separately.

PFC: prefrontal cortex. BF: basal forebrain. S: striatum. NA: nucleus accumbens. T: thalamus. Hy: hypothalamus. A: amygdala. H: hippocampus. NT: brain neurotransmitter center. SC: spinal cord. C: cerebellum.

Circuits and Symptoms in Depression, Part 1

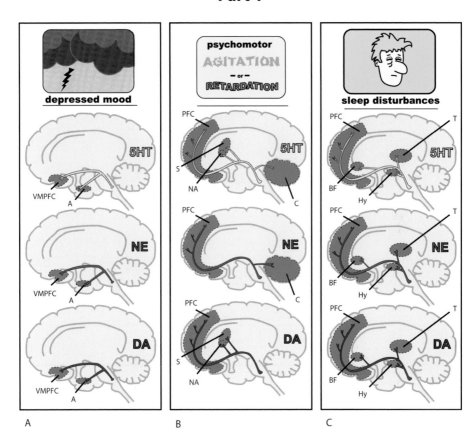

FIGURE 1.11.

A. Hypoactivation (denoted in blue) of serotonin (5HT), norepinephrine (NE), and/or dopamine (DA) projections to the amygdala (A) and ventromedial prefrontal cortex (VMPFC) is hypothetically involved in depressed mood.

B. Inefficient information processing in the prefrontal cortex (PFC; 5HT, NE, and DA projections), the cerebellum (C; 5HT and NE projections), and the striatum (S) and nucleus accumbens (NA; 5HT and DA projections) is hypothetically involved in psychomotor agitation or retardation.

C. Hypoactivation of 5HT, NE, and DA projections from brainstem nuclei to the hypothalamus (Hy), thalamus (T), basal forebrain (BF), and PFC is hypothetically involved in sleep disturbances.

Circuits and Symptoms in Depression, Part 2

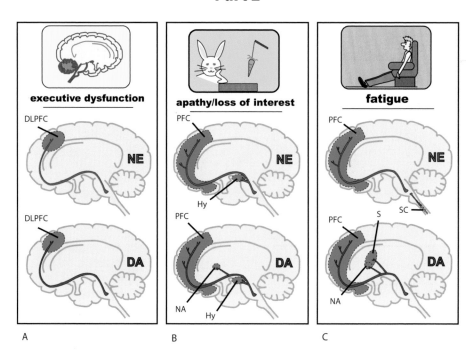

FIGURE 1.12.

A. Inefficient information processing from norepinephrine (NE) and dopamine (DA) projections to the dorsolateral prefrontal cortex (DLPFC) is hypothetically linked to problems with emotional regulation, self-monitoring, goal-setting, priority planning, and organization, all of which could lead to executive dysfunction.

B. Inefficient information processing from NE projections to the prefrontal cortex (PFC) and hypothalamus (Hy) and the DA projections to the PFC, Hy, and nucleus accumbens (NA) is hypothetically linked to apathy. Although superficially similar to depressed mood, apathy is actually a distinct symptom of depression, associated with lack of pleasure including decreased libido, linked to loss of interest and motivation, and often experienced by geriatric patients. Additionally, apathy is also hypothetically regulated by different brain circuits than depressed mood.

C. Inefficient information processing from NE and DA projections to the PFC is hypothetically involved in mental fatigue. Physical fatigue is linked to deficient NE functioning in the descending spinal cord and deficient DA functioning in the striatum, NA, Hy, and spinal cord.

Circuits and Symptoms in Depression, Part 3

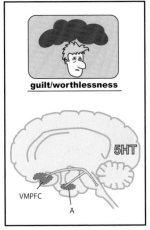

guilt/worthlessness

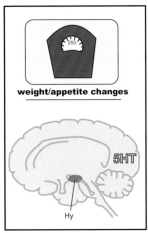

weight/appetite changes

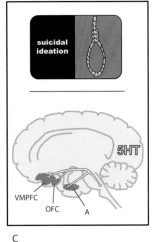

A   B   C

FIGURE 1.13.

A. Inefficient or dysfunctional serotonin (5HT) projections to the amygdala (A) and the ventromedial prefrontal cortex (VMPFC) could theoretically cause feelings of guilt and worthlessness, which are regulated by these "emotional" brain regions.

B. Inefficient or dysfunctional 5HT projections to the hypothalamus (Hy) could theoretically lead to problems with weight and appetite.

C. 5HT projections to the "emotional" brain regions including the amygdala (A), VMPFC, and orbital frontal cortex (OFC), could hypothetically be involved in suicidal ideation.

Circuits and Symptoms in Depression:
The Affect Meter

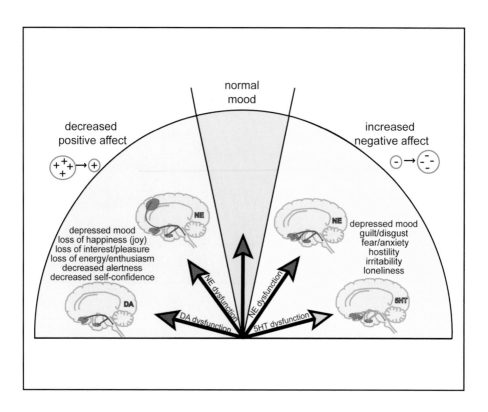

FIGURE 1.14. Depression comprises various mood-related symptoms that either represent decreased positive affect (on the left) or increased negative affect (on the right). A reduction in positive affect can lead to the symptoms on the left half of the affect-meter, with dopaminergic (DA) and noradrenergic (NE) dysfunction hypothetically playing a role. Heightened negative affect may lead to the symptoms on the right half of the affect-meter with theoretical serotonergic (5HT) and noradrenergic (NE) dysfunction.

Circuits in Mania

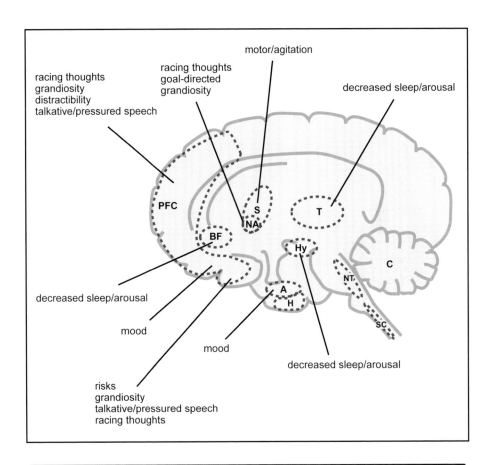

FIGURE 1.15. Various brain regions are hypothetically associated with particular symptom(s) of mania, and aberrant neuronal activity in any of these regions can theoretically lead to symptoms of acute mania. The following several pages examine each of these symptoms and regions separately.

PFC: prefrontal cortex. BF: basal forebrain. S: striatum. NA: nucleus accumbens. T: thalamus. Hy: hypothalamus. A: amygdala. H: hippocampus. NT: brain neurotransmitter center. SC: spinal cord. C: cerebellum.

Circuits and Symptoms in Mania, Part 1

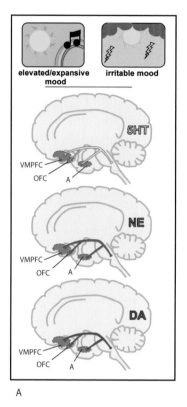

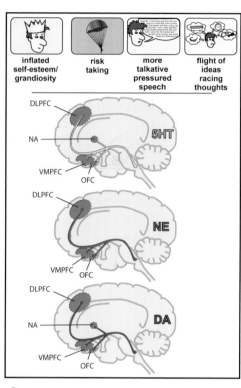

A

B

FIGURE 1.16.

A. Hyperactivity (denoted in red) of serotonin (5HT), norepinephrine (NE), and dopamine (DA) projections to the amygdala (A), ventromedial prefrontal cortex (VMPFC), and orbital frontal cortex (OFC), can hypothetically lead to symptoms of elevated/expansive or irritable mood.

B. Hyperactivity of 5HT and DA projections to the nucleus accumbens (NA), the region also implicated in the positive symptoms of psychosis, can hypothetically lead to symptoms of grandiosity and flight of ideas. Risk taking and garrulousness, which might be manifestations of poor impulse control, are hypothesized to be associated with 5HT, NE, and DA hyperactivity in the OFC. These four symptoms are also thought to have some association with the dorsolateral prefrontal cortex (DLPFC) and VMPFC.

Circuits and Symptoms in Mania, Part 2

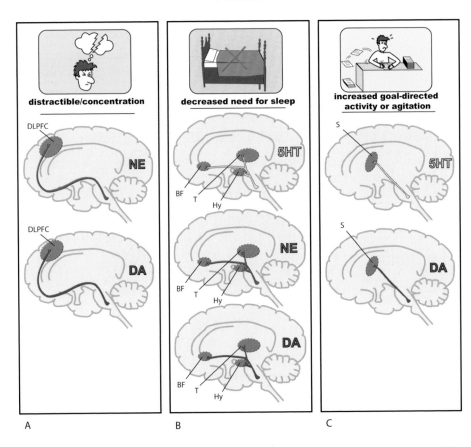

distractible/concentration

decreased need for sleep

increased goal-directed activity or agitation

DLPFC — NE

DLPFC — DA

5HT — BF, T, Hy

NE — BF, T, Hy

DA — BF, T, Hy

S — 5HT

S — DA

A

B

C

FIGURE 1.17.

A. Hyperactivity of norepinephrine (NE) and dopamine (DA) projections to the dorsolateral prefrontal cortex (DLPFC) might be associated with cognitive problems in mania such as poor concentration and/or distractibility.

B. Serotonin (5HT), NE, and DA projections to the thalamus (T), hypothalamus (Hy), and basal forebrain (BF) hypothetically regulate sleep in mania as well as depression, though inefficient information processing in mania hypothetically leads to reduced "need" for sleep while insomnia or hypersomnia is generally manifested in depression.

C. Hyperactive 5HT and DA projections to the striatum (S) are hypothetically associated with increased goal-directed activity or agitation in mania.

Bipolar Storm:
Unstable and Excessive Neurotransmission

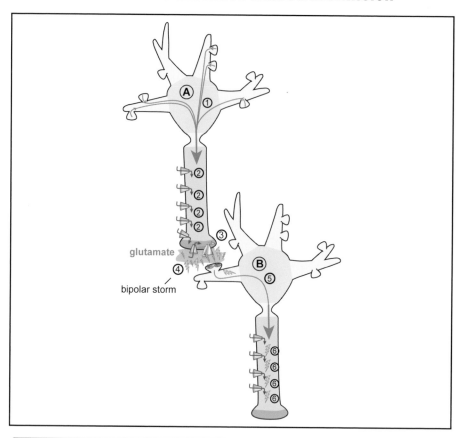

FIGURE 1.18. Bipolar disorder may be a result of unstable and excessive neuro-transmission, rather than resulting from a mixture of hyper- and hypoactive circuits. This figure illustrates such activity as a "bipolar storm" that culminates at synapses. Neuron A is hyperactive because widespread input from its dendritic tree (1) triggers too much axonal impulse flow via voltage-sensitive sodium channels (2). This nerve impulse hyperactivates voltage-sensitive calcium channels linked to glutamate release (3), thus triggering the "bipolar storm" (4) of excessive, chaotic, or unpredict-able neurotransmission from neuron A to neuron B. Postsynaptic N-methyl-d-aspar-tate (NMDA) receptors on neuron B detect this bipolar storm (4), and propagate the excessive, chaotic, or unpredictable neurotransmission to neuron B (5), which in turn converts this information into its own heightened nerve impulse, its own excessive activation of voltage-sensitive sodium channels (6), and so on.

Chapter 2

Neurobiology of Schizophrenia

Chapter 2 aims to describe the hypothetical neurobiology of schizophrenia thought to underlie the symptoms of the disorder. The dopamine hypothesis of schizophrenia has been accepted for a long time, especially as the first antipsychotics were shown to block dopamine D2 receptors. In addition, theories about the involvement of glutamate and serotonin have gained momentum in the pathophysiology of schizophrenia. This chapter will show that schizophrenia does not necessarily result from a hypo- or hyperactive dopamine system, but that it might be more accurate to say that dopamine is "out of tune." Additionally, this chapter will give a brief overview on how these three neurotransmitter systems may converge to induce both the positive and negative symptoms of schizophrenia.

Key Dopamine Pathways

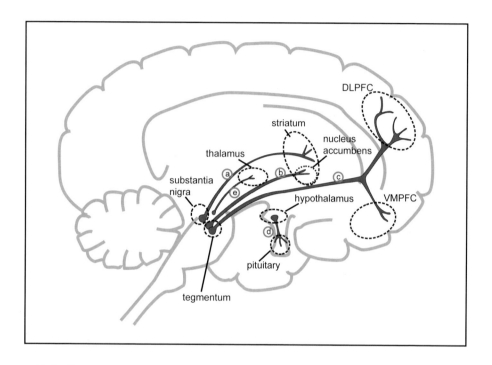

FIGURE 2.1. Five dopamine (DA) pathways are relevant in explaining the symptoms of schizophrenia and the therapeutic and side effects of antipsychotic drugs. **(a)** The nigrostriatal DA pathway is part of the extrapyramidal nervous system, which controls motor function and movement. **(b)** The mesolimbic DA pathway is part of the brain's limbic system, which regulates behaviors including pleasurable sensations, the powerful euphoria of drugs of abuse, and the delusions and hallucinations seen in psychosis. **(c)** The mesocortical DA pathway is implicated in mediating the cognitive symptoms (dorsolateral prefrontal cortex, DLPFC) and affective symptoms (ventromedial prefrontal cortex, VMPFC) of schizophrenia. **(d)** The tuberoinfundibular DA pathway projects from the hypothalamus to the anterior pituitary gland and controls prolactin secretion. **(e)** The fifth DA pathway arises from multiple sites, including the periaqueductal gray, ventral mesencephalon, hypothalamic nuclei, and lateral parabrachial nucleus and projects to the thalamus. Its function is not well known.

Key Glutamate Pathways

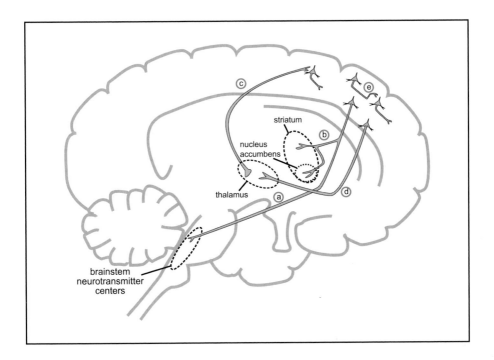

FIGURE 2.2. Similarly to dopamine (DA), there are five glutamate pathways in the brain that are of particular relevance to schizophrenia. **(a)** The cortical brainstem glutamate projection descends from layer 5 pyramidal neurons in the prefrontal cortex to brainstem neurotransmitter centers, including the raphe (serotonin), the locus coeruleus (norepinephrine), and the ventral tegmental area and substantia nigra (DA). This projection mainly regulates neurotransmitter release in the brainstem. **(b)** The cortico-striatal glutamate pathway descends from the prefrontal cortex to the striatum and the cortico-accumbens glutamate pathway sends projections to the nucleus accumbens. These pathways make up the "cortico-striatal" portion of cortico-striatal-thalamic loops. **(c)** Thalamo-cortical glutamate pathways encompass pathways ascending from the thalamus and innervating pyramidal neurons in the cortex. **(d)** Cortico-thalamic glutamate pathways descend from the PFC to the thalamus. **(e)** The cortico-cortical glutamatergic pathways allow intracortical pyramidal neurons to communicate with each other.

The Dopamine Hypothesis of Schizophrenia: Positive Symptoms

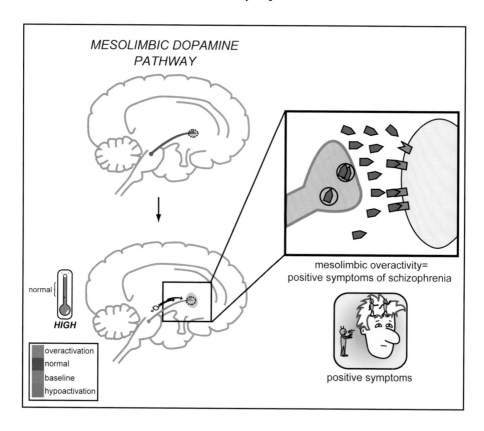

FIGURE 2.3. The mesolimbic dopamine (DA) pathway sends DA projections from cell bodies in the ventral tegmental area to the nucleus accumbens in the ventral striatum. This pathway hypothetically regulates emotional behaviors, pleasure, and reward and is the main candidate thought to regulate the positive symptoms of psychosis. Specifically, it has been hypothesized that hyperactivity of this pathway accounts for the delusions and hallucinations observed in schizophrenia. This hypothesis is known both as the "DA hypothesis of schizophrenia" and perhaps more precisely as the "mesolimbic DA hyperactivity hypothesis of positive symptoms of schizophrenia."

The Dopamine Hypothesis of Schizophrenia: Negative, Cognitive, and Affective Symptoms

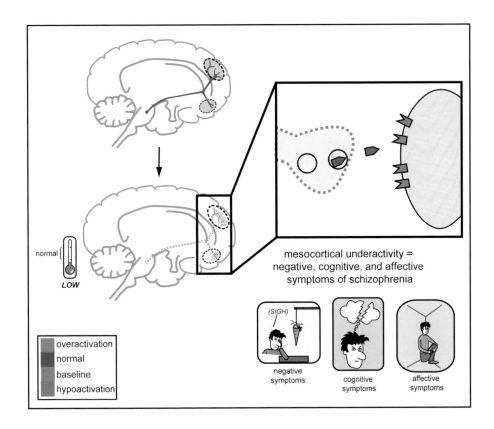

FIGURE 2.4. The mesocortical dopamine (DA) pathway is hypothetically also affected in schizophrenia. Here, DA cell bodies in the ventral tegmental area send projections to the dorsolateral prefrontal cortex (DLPFC) to regulate cognition and executive functions, and to the ventromedial prefrontal cortex (VMPFC) to regulate emotions and affect. Hypoactivation of this pathway theoretically results in the negative, cognitive, and affective symptoms seen in schizophrenia. This hypothesis is sometimes called the "mesocortical DA hypoactivity hypothesis of negative, cognitive, and affective symptoms" of schizophrenia. This DA deficit could result from ongoing degeneration due to glutamate excitotoxicity or from a neurodevelopmental impairment in the glutamatergic system. Loss of motivation and interest, anhedonia, and lack of pleasure as observed in schizophrenia result not only from a malfunctioning mesocortical DA pathway but also from a deficient mesolimbic DA pathway.

The Integrated Dopamine
Hypothesis of Schizophrenia

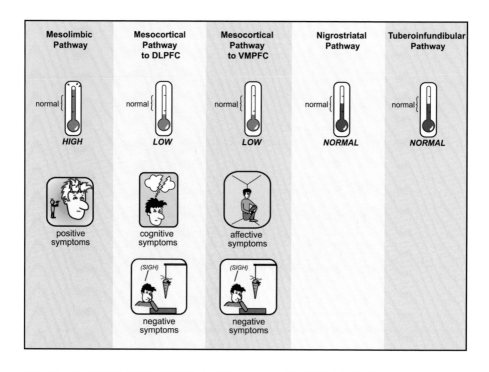

FIGURE 2.5. In schizophrenia, it appears that some dopamine (DA) pathways are overactive (mesolimbic pathway), others underactive (mesocortical pathway), and others are functioning normally (nigrostriatal and tuberoinfundibular pathway). Thus the DA system is neither "all too high" nor "all too low" but more precisely "out of tune," and DA needs to be increased in some areas, decreased in others, and left untouched in yet another set of circuits. Various antipsychotic drugs acting at different receptor subtypes, especially blocking D2 receptors and serotonin 2A (5HT2A) receptors, might lead to that outcome. Alternatively, regulating DA output by modulating transmitters such as glutamate may prove to be another way to "normalize" or "tune" DA circuits.

NMDA Receptor Hypofunction
Hypothesis of Schizophrenia

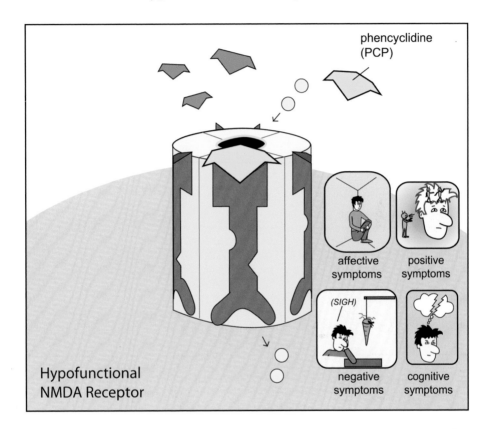

FIGURE 2.6. The NMDA (N-methyl-d-aspartate) receptor hypofunction hypothesis has been put forth in an attempt to explain mesolimbic dopamine (DA) hyperactivity. This hypothesis relies on the observation that when normal humans ingest phencyclidine (PCP), an NMDA receptor antagonist, they experience positive symptoms very similar to those observed in schizophrenia such as hallucinations and delusions. Thus hypoactive glutamate NMDA receptors could theoretically explain the biological basis for the mesolimbic DA hyperactivity. PCP also induces affective symptoms such as blunted affect, negative symptoms such as social withdrawal, and cognitive symptoms such as executive dysfunction in normal humans. Hypofunctional NMDA receptors might therefore be involved in all symptoms of schizophrenia.

Role of Glutamate in Schizophrenia

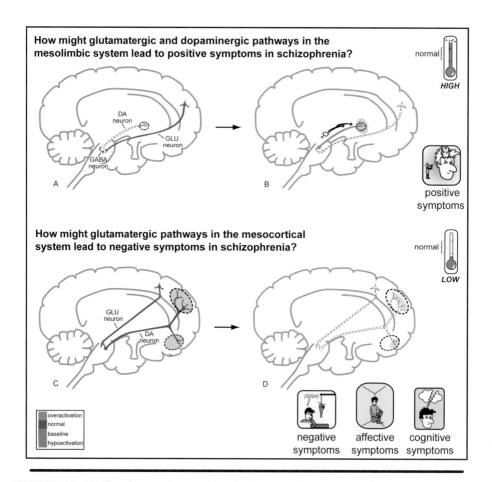

FIGURE 2.7. (A) The descending cortico-brainstem glutamate pathway normally leads to tonic inhibition of the mesolimbic dopamine (DA) pathway, via gamma-aminobutyric acid (GABA) interneurons in the ventral tegmental area. (B) When glutamate projections become hypoactive, this tonic inhibition is hypothetically missing, leading to hyperactivity of the mesolimbic DA pathway, which could be one theory explaining the overactivity of the mesolimbic DA pathway in schizophrenia. (C) In the ventral tegmental area, the cortico-brainstem glutamate projections can also directly synapse onto DA neurons, thus tonically exciting the mesocortical DA pathway. (D) Hypoactivity in glutamate projections, similarly to what is observed following phencyclidine administration can thus theoretically result in lost activation of the mesocortical DA neurons and might be the cause of the negative, cognitive, and affective symptoms seen in schizophrenia.

Opposing Actions of 5HT1A and 5HT2A Receptors on Dopamine Release

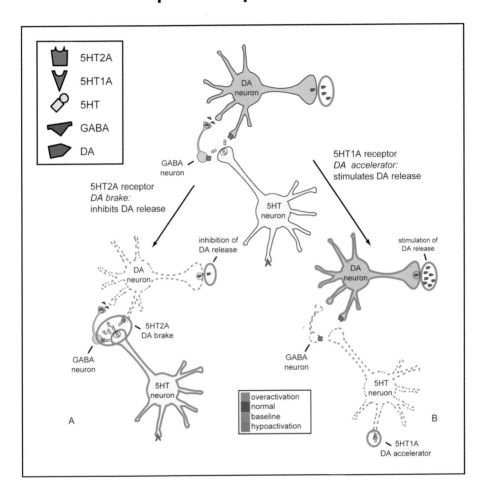

FIGURE 2.8. Serotonin (5HT) neurons can act on somatodendritic regions of dopamine (DA) neurons. Specifically, 5HT1A and 5HT2A receptors have opposite actions on DA release. Stimulation of 5HT1A receptors increases DA release, and thus 5HT1A receptors act as a DA accelerator. Stimulation of 5HT2A receptors inhibits DA release; thus 5HT2A receptors act as a DA brake. 5HT can regulate DA release directly or indirectly. (A) When 5HT binds to 5HT2A receptors on DA neurons or on GABA neurons, DA release is decreased directly or via inhibition through GABA release, respectively. (B) Upon binding to 5HT1A receptors, 5HT causes inhibition of its own release. A lack of 5HT results in disinhibition of DA release, and therefore increased DA output.

Somatodendritic Blockade of 5HT2A
Receptors Leads to Increased Dopamine Release

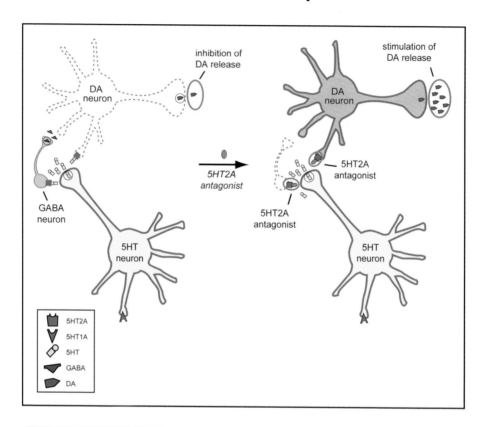

FIGURE 2.9. If stimulation of 5HT2A receptors leads to decreased dopamine (DA) release, then blocking 5HT2A receptors via antagonists should result in increased DA release. Increasing DA release can therefore be obtained by either blocking 5HT2A receptors on postsynaptic DA neurons or by blocking 5HT2A receptors on GABA interneurons.

Regulation of Dopamine Release by Serotonin in the Nigrostriatal Pathway: Parts 1 and 2

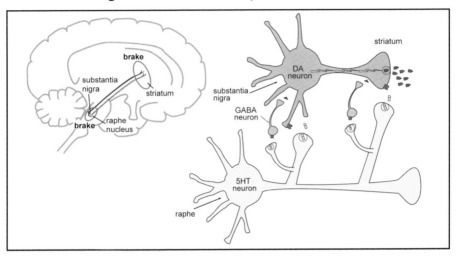

FIGURE 2.10. In the nigrostriatal pathway, the serotonin (5HT)-dopamine (DA) interaction mediates extrapyramidal side effects. Here 5HT can regulate DA release by acting on the somatodendritic regions of the DA neuron in the substantia nigra, or by acting on the axonal regions of the DA neuron in the striatum. Part 1: In the absence of 5HT, DA is freely released in the striatum.

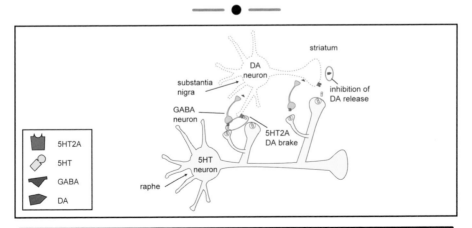

FIGURE 2.11. Part 2: When 5HT is released from raphe projections to the substantia nigra (red circle on the left), it stimulates postsynaptic somatodendritic 5HT2A receptors on DA and GABA neurons. This will lead to inhibition of axonal DA release (red circle on the right).

Regulation of Dopamine Release by Serotonin in the Nigrostriatal Pathway: Parts 3 and 4

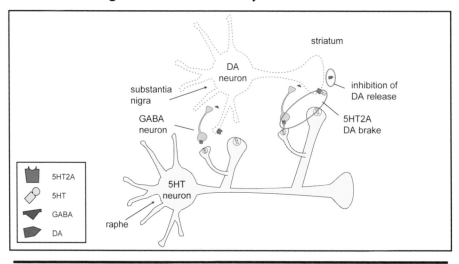

FIGURE 2.12. Part 3: When serotonin (5HT) is released from a synaptic connection projecting from axoaxonal contacts or by volume neurotransmission between 5HT and dopamine (DA) axon terminals (red circle, bottom), it will stimulate postsynaptic 5HT2A receptors on DA and GABA neurons, leading to decreased axonal DA release (red circle, top).

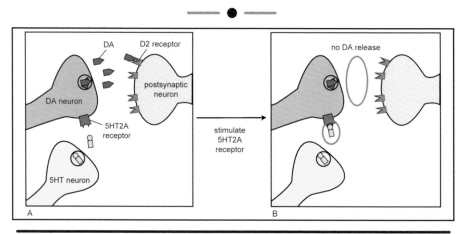

FIGURE 2.13. Part 4: At the level of striatal axons, 5HT normally inhibits DA release. (A) In the absence of 5HT, however, DA is released without hindrance. (B) In the presence of 5HT, 5HT2A receptors on DA terminals are stimulated, thus inhibiting DA release, thereby leading to a lack of synaptic DA.

Serotonin Also Modulates Cortical Glutamate Release

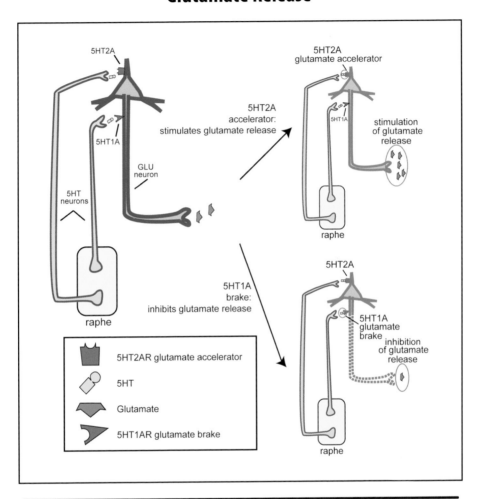

FIGURE 2.14. Stimulation of 5HT2A and 5HT1A receptors also leads to an opposing modulation of cortical glutamate release, but does so contrary to the actions of these same serotonin (5HT) receptors upon dopamine (DA) release. Here, stimulation of 5HT2A receptors located on glutamate cell bodies induces an increase in glutamate release, acting as a glutamate accelerator. Stimulation of 5HT1A receptors located on glutamate axons inhibits glutamate release, acting as a glutamate brake. This is contrary to the regulation that 5HT has on DA release (see Figure 2.8) where stimulation of 5HT2A receptors leads to inhibition of DA release (brake) and stimulation of 5HT1A receptors leads to increased DA release (accelerator).

Strengthening the Signal-to-Noise Ratio in Schizophrenia

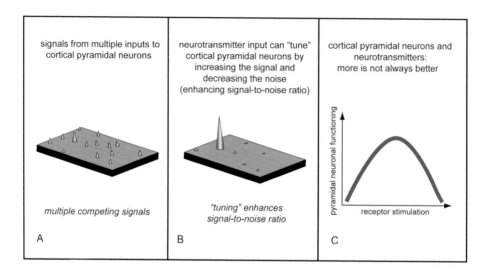

FIGURE 2.15. (A) Adequate information processing occurs when all neurotransmitters are working in tune. In schizophrenia, however, information processing in specific key brain areas is abnormal. Prefrontal cortical activity in schizophrenia is not just "too high" or "too low," but it is most likely "out of tune" or "chaotic," with some areas hyperactive and others hypoactive. (B) When prefrontal neurons are adequately tuned, the signal-to-noise ratio is sensitive enough to allow for proper filtering of "noise," resulting in the strengthening of one signal over another. (C) As represented by the inverted U-shaped curve, moderation is preferable when it comes to receptor stimulation. Too much or too little stimulation is suboptimal. Thus in order to reach the optimal tuning of the signal-to-noise ratio it is important to determine where the system is on the curve, as it might need to be either increased or decreased.

Chapter 3

Lithium and Other Anticonvulsants for the Treatment of Bipolar Disorders

Chapter 3 aims to describe the complex pharmacology of mood stabilizers used to treat bipolar disorders. Additionally, this chapter aims to recognize how different mood stabilizing drugs affect the various disease states of bipolar disorder and to identify mechanisms as well as therapeutic benefits and nuances of drugs commonly prescribed for bipolar disorder.

This chapter introduces pharmacologic mechanisms of action of some of the major mood-stabilizing drugs used in the treatment of bipolar disorder. By combining knowledge of symptoms and neurobiology from previous chapters, it becomes clear how these medications can potentially help treat some of the malfunctioning brain circuits in bipolar disorder. This chapter will introduce a few specific compounds of this class of medications.

Mood Stabilizer Biology:
Voltage-sensitive Sodium Channels

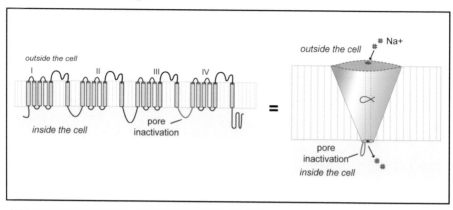

FIGURE 3.1. Ion channels that open and close in response to the charge or voltage across the membrane are called "voltage-sensitive" or "voltage-gated." Four subunits (on the left) combine to form the alpha pore subunit, or channel, for sodium in a voltage-sensitive sodium channel (VSSC; on the right).

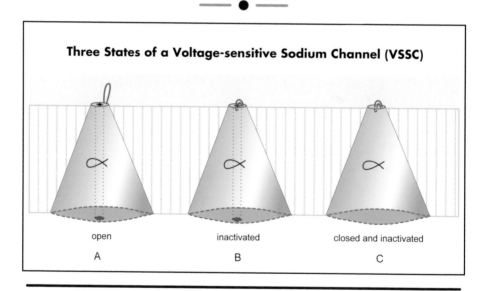

FIGURE 3.2. Voltage-sensitive sodium channels (VSSCs) are involved in neurotransmission via sodium influx and exist in three different states: they can be opened, allowing ions to flow through the channel (A), they can be inactivated, rapidly preventing ion flow (B), or they can be closed and inactivated, more stably preventing ion flow (C).

Mood Stabilizer Biology:
Voltage-sensitive Calcium Channels

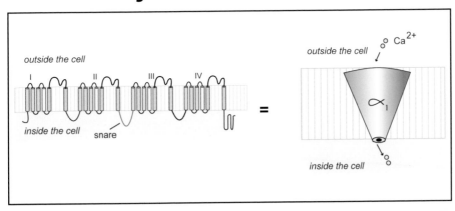

FIGURE 3.3. Four subunits (on the left) combine to form the alpha 1 pore subunit, or channel, for calcium in a voltage-sensitive calcium channel (VSCC; on the right).

— ● —

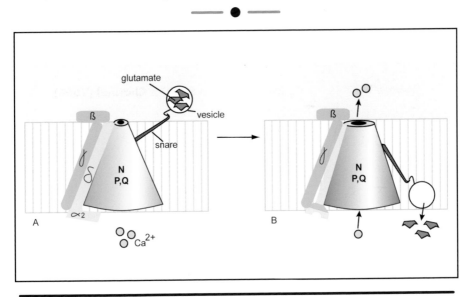

FIGURE 3.4. VSCCs regulate neurotransmission through the use of a "snare" protein mechanism. (A) The snare, which is made up of intracellular amino acids that link the second to the third subunits of the alpha 1 unit, holds on to a synaptic vesicle, here filled with glutamate. (B) When an electrical impulse arrives, the presynaptic N or P/Q calcium channel opens to allow calcium flow, and the snare "fires" and causes neurotransmitter release.

Voltage-sensitive Sodium and Calcium Channels Regulate Signal Propagation

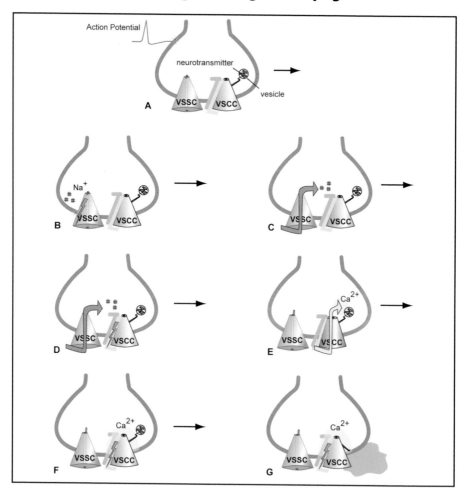

FIGURE 3.5. Voltage-sensitive sodium and calcium channels work together to produce neurotransmission, a process known as excitation-secretion coupling. Voltage-sensitive sodium channels (VSSCs) detect an action potential and send the signal along the axon via sodium release (A). The released sodium triggers the opening of the VSSCs at the axon terminal (B). Sodium comes into the presynaptic neuron (C) where it changes the electrical charge of the voltage-sensitive calcium channel (VSCC; D), opening it and allowing calcium into the neuron (E). The calcium concentration increases (F), causing synaptic vesicles to merge with the presynaptic membrane, leading to neurotransmitter release (G).

Anti-manic Action at Voltage-sensitive Sodium Channels

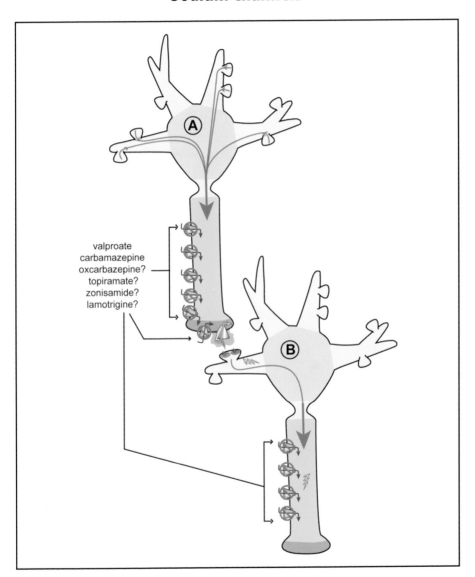

FIGURE 3.6. Bipolar disorder may ultimately result from unstable and excessive neurotransmission culminating in the "bipolar storm" (see Figure 1.18). Drugs such as valproate, carbamazepine, oxcarbazepine, topimarate, zonisamide, and lamotrigine may theoretically exert stabilizing effects on neurotransmission.

Lithium: Possible Mechanisms of Action on Downstream Signal Transduction Cascades

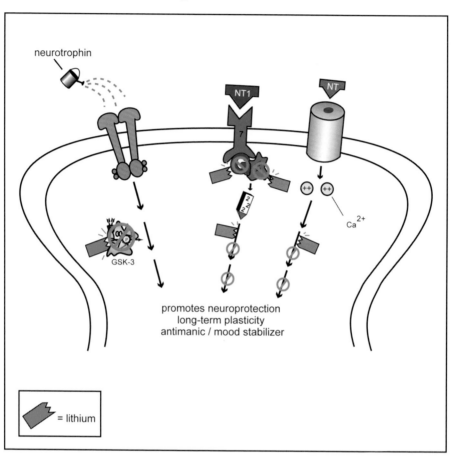

FIGURE 3.7. Although the mechanisms of action of lithium are still not completely known, they are posited to include modulating G proteins (middle) or inhibiting second messenger enzymes such as inositol monophosphatase, which can affect signal transduction for neurotransmission not only at G protein-linked receptors (middle) but also at ion channel-linked receptors (right). Lithium might also act within various downstream signal transduction cascades for neurotrophic factors (left).

In terms of treatment benefits, lithium's efficacy has been better established for treating and preventing mania rather than depression. Unfortunately, it may be less effective for rapid cycling or mixed episodes. It has, however, proven efficacious at preventing suicide.

Valproate:
Possible Sites of Action on Signal Cascades

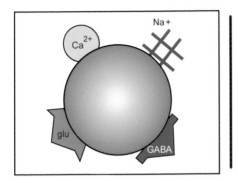

FIGURE 3.8. While the actual mechanism of action of **valproate** in bipolar disorder remains unknown, it is known that valproate has downstream effects on signal transduction cascades. Valproate is approved for use in bipolar disorder and also as an anticonvulsant.

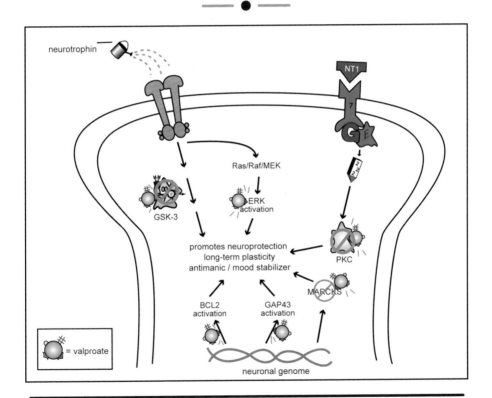

FIGURE 3.9. Valproate may inhibit signals that modulate synaptic function in nerve terminals and activate signals that promote neuroprotection and long-term plasticity. Valproate has nonspecific actions on GABA, as well as nonspecific actions at voltage-sensitive sodium and calcium channels.

Valproate: Possible Sites of Action on GABA and Voltage-sensitive Sodium Channels

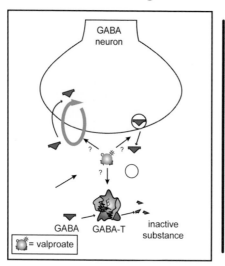

FIGURE 3.10. Valproate's effects on GABA are nonspecific and might involve inhibiting reuptake, enhancing release, or interfering with metabolism. Enhancing GABA neurotransmission might reduce manic symptoms.

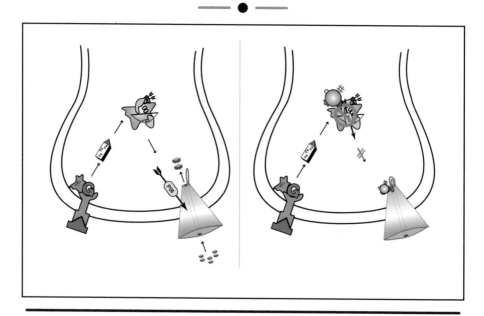

FIGURE 3.11. Valproate might directly bind to specific subunits of sodium channels, or it might inhibit phosphorylating enzymes that modulate sodium channel sensitivity. The inhibition of sodium channels can lead to reduced sodium influx which could, by decreasing glutamate excitatory neurotransmission, modulate manic symptoms.

Carbamazepine, Oxcarbazepine, and Eslicarbazepine

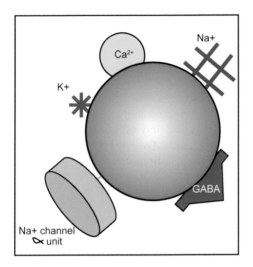

Carbamazepine is effective at treating mania and may be effective at preventing manic episodes. Its efficacy in treating or preventing depression is not well established. Carbamazepine has multiple mechanisms of action including modulation of GABA and sodium, calcium, and potassium ion channels, with a particular site of action on the alpha unit of sodium channels. Carbamazepine is approved for epilepsy and bipolar mania (the XR formulation), and it is commonly prescribed for bipolar depression, bipolar maintenance, and is often used as an adjunct in the treatment of psychosis and schizophrenia.

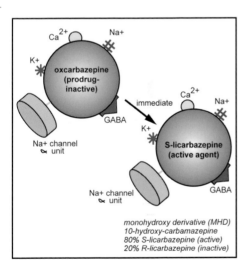

Despite their similarity to carbamazepine, the mood-stabilizing effects of **oxcarbazepine** and **eslicarbazepine** have not been established. Oxcarbazepine is an inactive compound (prodrug). It is converted into two enantiomers (R and S) of the 10-hydroxy derivative monohydroxy-derivative, which is called licarbazepine; the S enantiomer is the active form of this drug, also called eslicarbazepine. The active eslicarbazepine itself is in testing as a possible mood stabilizer since oxcarbazepine has never been approved for this use. Oxcarbazepine is an approved anticonvulsant.

FIGURE 3.12. Properties of carbamazepine, oxcarbazepine, and eslicarbazepine.

Lamotrigine and Riluzole

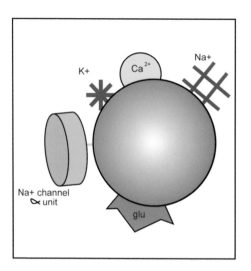

Lamotrigine's mechanisms of action include modulation of glutamate as well as sodium, calcium, and potassium ion channels, with a particular site of action on the alpha unit of sodium channels. Lamotrigine is approved for bipolar I maintenance and for partial seizures. As it has proven efficacious at treating bipolar depression and preventing the recurrence of both manic and depressive episodes, it is often prescribed for these states. It is also prescribed for psychosis and schizophrenia.

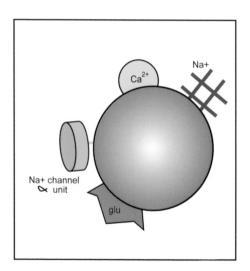

Riluzole has hypothetical actions on glutamate and on sodium, calcium, and potassium ion channels, with a particular site of action on the alpha unit of sodium channels. Riluzole is an approved treatment for amyotrophic lateral sclerosis (ALS), where it works presumably by reducing glutamate release and thus glutamate-mediated excitotoxicity. Riluzole also has anticonvulsant actions and may also be effective in bipolar disorder as its mechanisms of action appear similar to lamotrigine (i.e., blocking alpha subunit of voltage-sensitive sodium channels and reducing excitatory glutamate neurotransmission). Riluzole is often prescribed for treatment-resistant cases of bipolar and unipolar depression, even though it is not approved for such uses.

FIGURE 3.13. Properties of lamotrigine and riluzole.

Agents with Binding Sites on Voltage-sensitive Sodium Channels

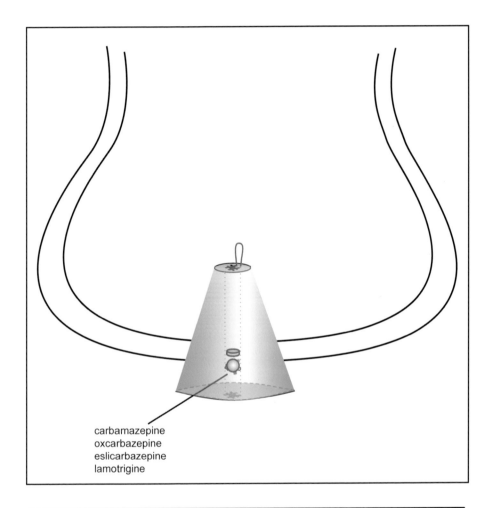

carbamazepine
oxcarbazepine
eslicarbazepine
lamotrigine

FIGURE 3.14. Carbamazepine and eslicarbazepine are thought to share a common binding site on the alpha subunit of voltage-sensitive sodium channels (VSSCs). They are thought to effectively reduce manic symptoms by binding to the open channel conformation, interfering with the conductance of sodium ions through VSSCs. These drugs may also increase GABA neurotransmission, enhancing its inhibitory properties.

Riluzole and Lamotrigine:
Possible Sites of Action on Glutamate

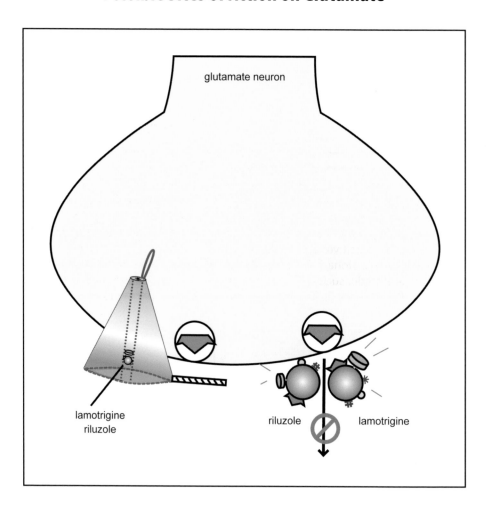

FIGURE 3.15. Lamotrigine also acts through a yet unknown mechanism to reduce excitatory glutamate neurotransmission. Similarly to riluzole, lamotrigine may reduce glutamate neurotransmission through actions on voltage-sensitive sodium channels (VSSCs, left) or through as-yet-undefined synaptic actions (right). Modulation of glutamatergic neurotransmission may be related to the efficacy of these compounds to relieve the symptoms of mania.

Gabapentin and Pregabalin and Their Molecular Actions

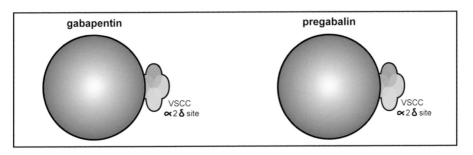

FIGURE 3.16. Gabapentin and pregabalin are anticonvulsants approved for neuropathic pain (both), fibromyalgia (pregabalin), and anxiety (pregabalin, in Europe). They are not, however, approved for bipolar disorder. These agents have a mechanism of action different from other known mood stabilizers. As they bind to the alpha 2 delta subunit of voltage-sensitive calcium channels (VSCCs), they are often referred to as alpha 2 delta ligands. Alpha 2 delta ligands may be helpful in treating ancillary symptoms of bipolar disorder such as sleep disturbances and anxiety, but most studies fail to show robust mood-stabilizing actions on either mania or depression.

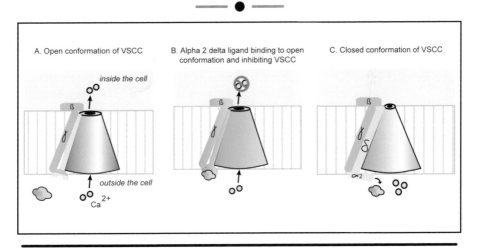

FIGURE 3.17. Calcium influx occurs when voltage-sensitive calcium channels (VSCCs) are in the open channel conformation (A). Alpha 2 delta ligands such as gabapentin and pregabalin have the greatest affinity for the open channel conformation and thus block the channels that are most active (B), thereby decreasing glutamate release. Alpha 2 delta ligands do not bind to the closed conformation of VSCCs, and thus do not disrupt normal neurotransmission (C).

Topiramate, Zonisamide, and Levetiracetam

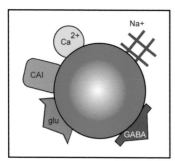

Topiramate has possible pharmacological actions on glutamate and GABA and on sodium and calcium channels. It is also a weak carbonic anhydrase inhibitor, but its exact binding site is not known. It has been tested in bipolar disorder with varying results. It may help to reduce weight gain caused by other mood stabilizers. Topiramate is approved as an anticonvulsant and for migraines. Topiramate is commonly prescribed as an adjunctive treatment for bipolar disorder.

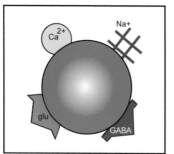

Zonisamide has possible actions on glutamate and GABA, presumably via actions on sodium and calcium channels. Its exact mechanism of action is not known. It has not been well tested in the treatment of bipolar disorder, but it is an approved anticonvulsant. Zonisamide is commonly prescribed for bipolar disorder.

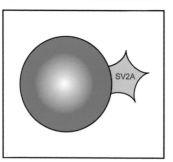

Levetiracetam has actions at SV2A proteins on synaptic vesicles, which are hypothesized to affect neurotransmitter release. Levetiracetam is an approved anticonvulsant but has not been well tested in the treatment of bipolar disorder, even though it is prescribed for mania.

FIGURE 3.18. Properties of topiramate, zonisamide, and levetiracetam.

Chapter 4

Antipsychotics for the Treatment of Bipolar Disorders and Schizophrenia

Chapter 4 aims to explain the complex pharmacology of antipsychotics and to recognize how different antipsychotic drugs affect the various symptoms of schizophrenia. Additionally, this chapter aims to recognize that side effects are linked to the drug's receptor profile.

The serendipitous discovery in the 1950s that the antihistamine chlorpromazine can relieve symptoms of psychosis led to the discovery of conventional antipsychotics. Their ability to block D2 receptors was recognized by the 1970s. Since then, much research has been done to improve antipsychotic medications. This chapter covers three topics: exploring the different classes of antipsychotics, elaborating on their properties, and describing the most common side effects of antipsychotics.

Conventional Antipsychotics
and Their Side Effects

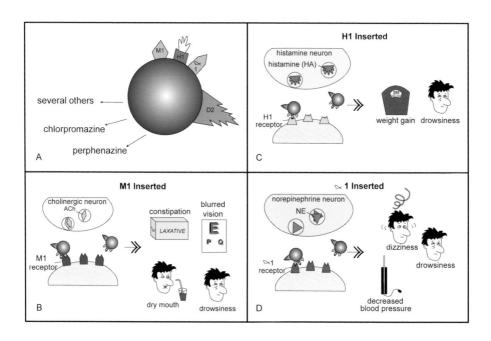

FIGURE 4.1. Conventional antipsychotics treat the symptoms of schizophrenia by blocking D2 receptors. Excessive blockade of D2 receptors, or blockade of DA receptors in hypoactive areas, can lead to many side effects, including "neurolepsis," an extreme form of slowness or absence of motor movement, as well as the worsening of negative, cognitive, and affective symptoms.

(A) Besides blockade at D2 receptors, conventional antipsychotics have additional pharmacologic properties: blockade of M1 muscarinic cholinergic receptors, H1 histamine receptors, and alpha1 adrenergic receptors. Medications with this receptor profile will exhibit similar side effects. (B) The M1 muscarinic anticholinergic portion of the drug can lead to constipation, blurred vision, dry mouth, and drowsiness when binding to acetylcholine receptors. (C) The H1 histamine portion of the drug can lead to drowsiness and weight gain. (D) The alpha 1 adrenergic portion of the drug can lead to dizziness, decreased blood pressure, and drowsiness.

Properties of Atypical Antipsychotics

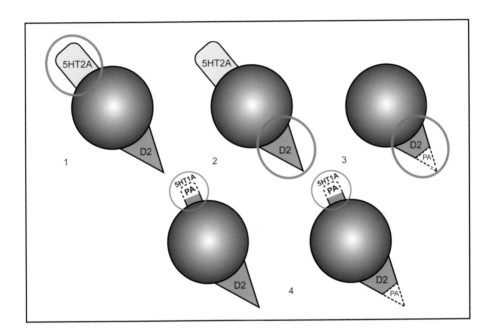

FIGURE 4.2. Atypical antipsychotics represent the second generation of antipsychotics. They are distinguished from conventional antipsychotics by their clinical properties (low extrapyramidal side effects and good efficacy for negative symptoms), as well as by four pharmacological characteristics: (1) Atypical antipsychotics couple their D2 antagonism with 5HT2A antagonism. (2) The dissociation rate at the D2 receptor sets apart the "atypicality" of an antipsychotic. Tight and long-lasting binding is characteristic of conventional antipsychotics, whereas rapid dissociation is a feature of atypical antipsychotics. (3) Atypical antipsychotics can also be D2 partial agonists (DPAs). These agents bind in a manner that is neither too antagonizing nor too stimulating, allowing for just the "right" amount of neurotransmission at D2 receptors. (4) Full or partial agonism at the 5HT1A receptor can also be a characteristic of some atypical antipsychotics. Stimulation at the 5HT1A receptor can increase dopamine release, thus improving affective, cognitive, and negative symptoms while reducing the risk of extrapyramidal side effects and prolactin elevation. Serotonin1A agonism can also decrease glutamate release, which may indirectly reduce the positive symptoms of psychosis.

Rapid Dissociation Theory of Atypical Antipsychotic Action

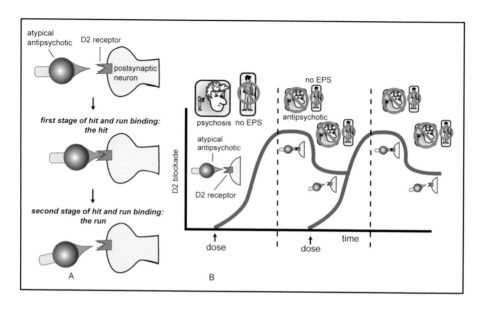

FIGURE 4.3. (A) Unlike conventional antipsychotics, atypical antipsychotics do not have "teeth" on their binding site, meaning that they cannot be locked into position upon binding to D2 receptors. Atypical antipsychotics interact loosely with D2 receptors, exemplified by their smooth binding site. This results in a rapid dissociation from the binding site, also referred to as the "hit and run" receptor binding property. Thus during the "hit," the atypical antipsychotic does not get locked into the receptor binding site and is able to "run" and slip away easily.

(B) An untreated patient with schizophrenia exhibits positive symptoms but no extrapyramidal side effects (EPS). Upon administration of an atypical antipsychotic, the D2 receptors get blocked for only a short period of time, in contrast to the long-lasting blockade from conventional antipsychotics. Only short blockade of D2 receptors is theoretically required for antipsychotic action, whereas persistent blockade of D2 receptors is required for EPS to occur. Atypical antipsychotics are beneficial in treating the positive symptoms of schizophrenia while preventing EPS, as dose after dose they bind just long enough to D2 receptors to induce antipsychotic effects, but they "run away" before eliciting EPS.

Conventional vs. Atypical Antipsychotics:
Part 1

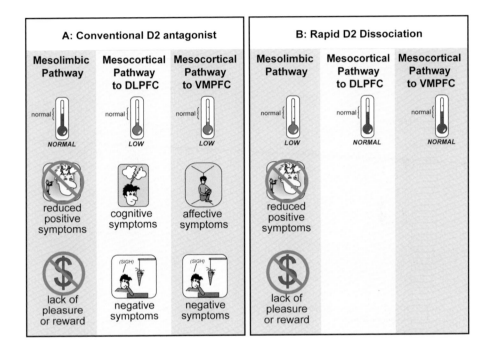

FIGURE 4.4. (A) A D2 antagonist reduces dopamine (DA) output indiscriminately throughout the brain. While positive symptoms of psychosis will be successfully reduced, the experience of pleasure also mediated by the mesolimbic DA pathway will be impaired. The near shut-down of the mesolimbic DA pathway necessary to improve positive symptoms can lead to anhedonia and apathy. Decreasing DA output in the hypoactive mesocortical pathways will further reduce this pathway's activity and can actually worsen cognitive, negative, or affective symptoms.

(B) Administration of an agent that rapidly dissociates from D2 receptors leads to a reduced DA output in the mesolimbic DA pathway, thus decreasing positive symptoms. Unfortunately, decreasing DA output in this pathway can also lower the experiences of pleasure and reward. Loose binding of atypical antipsychotics in the mesocortical DA pathway could potentially reset this pathway. Theoretically, persistent blockade of D2 receptors is needed in this pathway to worsen affective, cognitive, or negative symptoms. Thus rapid blockade of and dissociation from D2 receptors in the mesocortical pathway may not lead to these side effects.

Conventional vs. Atypical Antipsychotics: Part 2

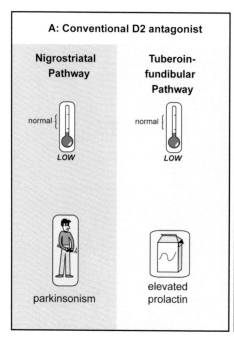

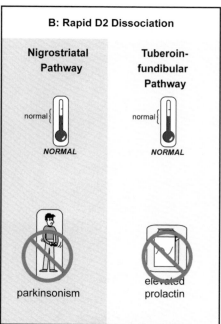

FIGURE 4.5. (A) By reducing dopamine (DA) output in the nigrostriatal pathway, D2 antagonists can lead to extrapyramidal side effects (EPS) and tardive dyskinesia. Chronic DA blockade of the tuberoinfundibular pathway will result in hyperprolactinemia and its accompanying complications.
(B) In the nigrostriatal and tuberoinfundibular DA pathways, administration of agents that rapidly dissociate from D2 receptors may exhibit reduced risk for EPS and may not lead to elevated prolactin levels, thus preventing some of the unwanted side effects inherent to conventional antipsychotics.

Atypical Antipsychotics:
Actions in Bipolar Depression

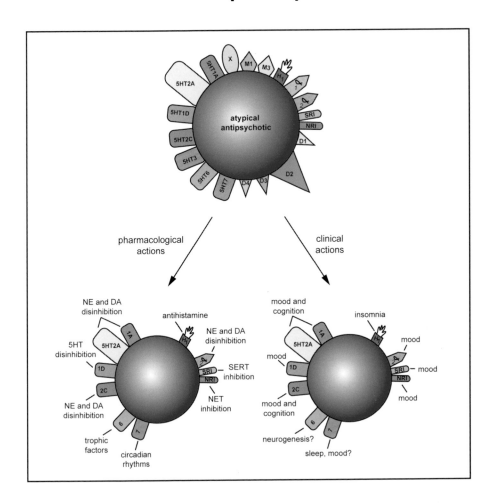

FIGURE 4.6. Atypical antipsychotics might relieve symptoms of bipolar depression by increasing availability of serotonin (5HT), norepinephrine (NE), and/or dopamine (DA) via various mechanisms of action as depicted in this figure. Each atypical agent has a different binding profile and therefore potentially different treatment capabilities.

Atypical Antipsychotics: Glutamate-reducing Actions in Psychotic and Nonpsychotic Mania

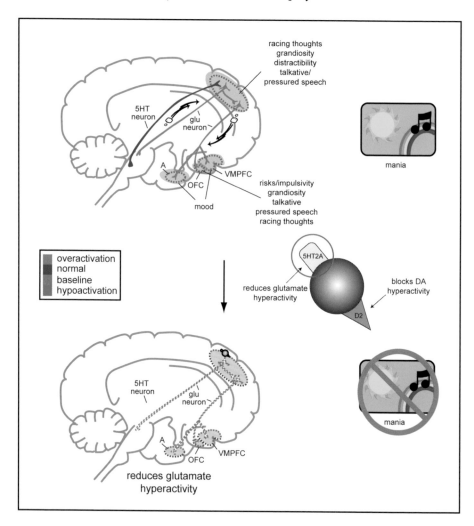

FIGURE 4.7. Glutamate hyperactivity may, through different pathways, contribute to the development of both manic and depressive symptoms in bipolar disorder. Atypical antipsychotics may alleviate symptoms of both psychotic and nonpsychotic mania as well as bipolar depression via 5HT2A antagonist properties. Blockade of 5HT2A receptors in the prefrontal cortex can lead to reduced glutamate hyperactivity, leading to decreased activity in the orbital frontal cortex (OFC) and ventromedial prefrontal cortex (VMPFC).

Atypical Antipsychotics: Dopamine-reducing Actions in Psychotic and Nonpsychotic Mania

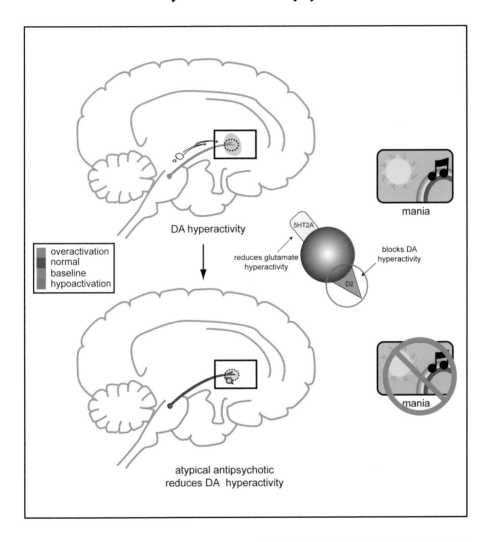

FIGURE 4.8. Dopamine (DA) hyperactivity could also play a role in the development of psychotic as well as nonpsychotic manic symptoms. Thus, reducing dopamine hyperactivity via D2 blockade by atypical antipsychotics may be an effective antimanic strategy.

The Agonist Spectrum:
The Theory Behind Partial Agonists

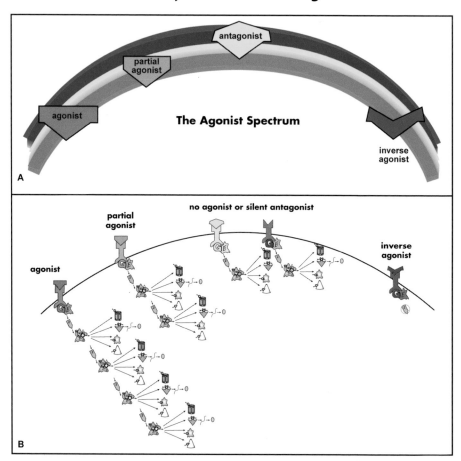

FIGURE 4.9. (A) Naturally occurring neurotransmitters, as well as drugs that stimulate receptors, are primary agonists. Drugs that stimulate a receptor to a lesser degree are partial agonists or stabilizers. Antagonists are "silent" and only block the action of agonists without having an action of their own. Inverse agonists can block the actions of the agonist, or they can reduce baseline activity in the absence of an agonist. (B) The concept of the agonist spectrum can also be adapted to the signal transduction system. A full agonist leads to maximal signal transduction; a partial agonist leads to a level of signal transduction between the full agonist and no agonist. Antagonists can only reduce the level of signal transduction caused by the agonist. Inverse agonists, on the other hand, can actually lead to lower levels of stimulation beyond what is normally produced in the absence of an agonist.

How Is the Dopamine Spectrum
Related to Receptor Output?

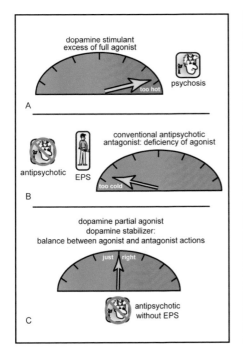

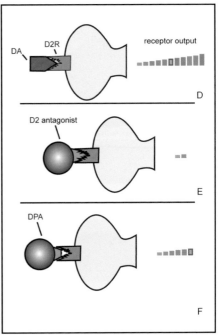

FIGURE 4.10. (Left) In order to understand the actions of dopamine (DA) and DA agents within an agonist spectrum, it may be helpful to look at them along a "hot-cold" spectrum. That is, DA acts as the ultimate agonist and is too "hot," resulting in psychosis (A). D2 blockers such as conventional antagonists are too "cold," and while they prevent psychotic episodes they also lead to extrapyramidal side effects (EPS) (B). Partial agonists are "lukewarm," leading to just the right stimulation of DA receptors, thus preventing psychotic episodes without inducing EPS (C).

(Right) In terms of output, DA is the ultimate full agonist, leading to full receptor output (D). At the other end of the spectrum, conventional antipsychotics (full antagonists) lead to only very little DA output (E). The atypical antipsychotics that have 5HT2A/D2 blocking activity lead to similarly little DA output. D2 partial agonists (DPAs), on the other hand, stimulate DA receptors only partially, leading to an intermediate or moderate DA output (F).

D2 and D3 Partial Agonists:
Overview

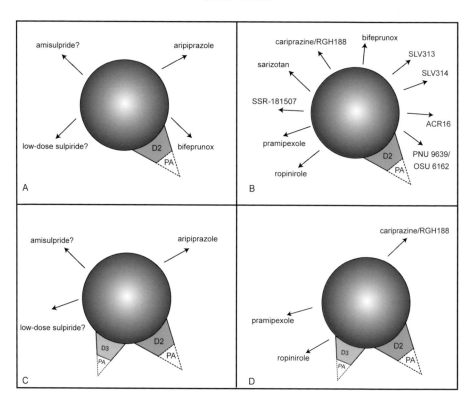

FIGURE 4.11. (A) There is currently only one well-established dopamine (DA) partial agonist on the market: aripiprazole. Bifeprunox is a DA partial agonist but was recently not approved by the FDA. Amisulpride and sulpiride are available outside the US and may act as partial agonists, particularly at low doses, but are not well characterized as DA partial agonists. (B) DA partial agonists currently in development include cariprazine/RGH188, bifeprunox, SLV313, SLV314, ACR16, SSR181507, and sarizotan. These agents are closer to the antagonist end of the partial agonist spectrum. D2 partial agonists that are closer to the full agonist end of the spectrum include pramipexole and ropinirole. These agents are in testing for bipolar depression and treatment-resistant depression but are not yet approved for these uses. (C and D) Often not emphasized in their pharmacologic characterization is the fact that most atypical antipsychotic agents act at D3 receptors, mostly as antagonists. Aripiprazole, however, acts as a D3 partial agonist. Amisulpride and sulpiride could also be D3 partial agonists. It is not clear what this action adds to D2 partial agonist action, but there is no selective D2 partial agonist nor any selective D3 partial agonist available.

5HT1A Partial Agonism
of Atypical Antipsychotics

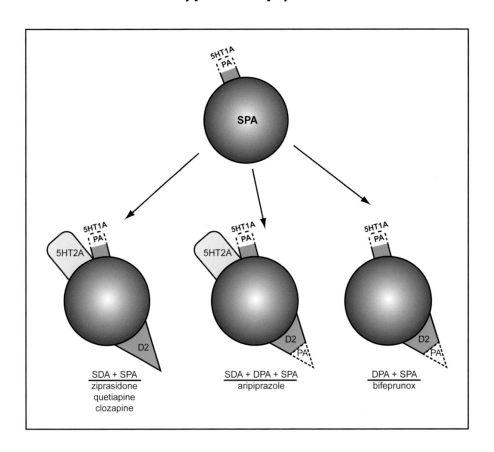

FIGURE 4.12. Various antipsychotics do not fit neatly into a single class of drugs because they combine different receptor actions. Besides being 5HT2A/D2 blockers, ziprasidone, quetiapine, and clozapine are also partial agonists at 5HT1A receptors. The D2 partial agonist aripiprazole is also an antagonist at 5HT2A receptors and a partial agonist at 5HT1A receptors. Besides being a D2 partial agonist, bifeprunox is also a partial agonist at the 5HT1A receptor. These additional properties are what make these compounds different from each other, and explains their different effectiveness in various individuals with specific ailments.

Properties of Atypical Antipsychotics: Part 1

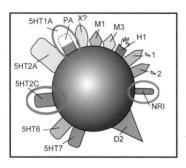

Quetiapine has widespread actions on serotonin (5HT), dopamine (DA), and norpeinephrine (NE) systems. Its active metabolite, norquetiapine, has unique features (red circles) that most likely add to quetiapine's efficacy. This very atypical antipsychotic exhibits rapid D2 dissociation, and therefore hardly any extrapyramidal side effects and no prolactin elevation. The partial 5HT1A agonist feature of quetiapine and the norepinephrine reuptake-inhibiting and 5HT2C blocking properties of norquetiapine are hypothetically responsible for its effectiveness at treating mood and cognitive disorders. Quetiapine is effective as a once-daily dose, and if given in the evening it will not induce daytime sedation. At moderate to high doses, both quetiapine and norquetiapine can induce weight gain due to histamine H1 blockade and 5HT2C blockade, respectively. Additionally, at these doses, quetiapine can increase triglyceride levels and insulin resistance, emphasizing the need to monitor patients if they are started on this atypical antipsychotic. Quetiapine is approved for the treatment of schizophrenia and the maintenance thereafter. It is also approved for acute mania and depressive episodes of bipolar disorder.

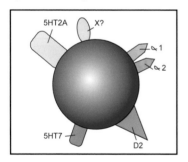

Risperidone has actions on 5HT, DA, and alpha 1 and 2 adrenergic receptors. Risperidone primarily functions as a 5HT2A/D2 antagonist; at low doses it behaves like an atypical antipsychotic, but if the dose is pushed it can lead to extrapyramidal side effects. Receptor "X" represents the unclear actions that some atypical antipsychotics have on the insulin system, where they change cellular insulin resistance and increase fasting plasma triglyceride levels. Risperidone is approved for use in children and adolescents for the following disorders: irritability associated with autistic disorder (ages 5 to 16), bipolar disorder (ages 10 to 17), and schizophrenia (ages 13 to 17). It is also approved for acute and mixed mania. Long-acting, two-week injectable risperidone, when added to other mood stabilizers, may delay relapse in patients with frequently relapsing bipolar disorder. Risperidone does increase prolactin levels, but there appears to be less risk of weight gain with risperidone, as well as less cardiometabolic risk than with some other atypical antipsychotics, at least in some patients.

FIGURE 4.13. Properties of some atypical antipsychotics: Part 1.

Properties of Atypical Antipsychotics: Part 2

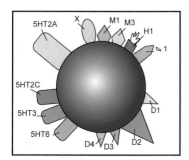

Olanzapine has widespread actions on serotonin (5HT) and dopamine (DA) systems and on muscarinic, histamine, and alpha 1 adrenergic receptors. It is one of the antipsychotics with the greatest cardiometabolic risk, as it leads to weight gain, increased fasting triglyceride levels, and increased insulin resistance. Olanzapine acts at numerous neurotransmitter receptors in addition to functioning as a 5HT2A/D2 antagonist. Olanzapine is often used at doses higher than what the packet insert suggests, as it often exhibits better efficacy and effectiveness at higher doses. Olanzapine appears to be effective at reducing affective and cognitive symptoms, a property most likely related in part to its 5HT2C antagonism. Its 5HT2C antagonist actions may contribute to its antidepressant effects, especially in combination with fluoxetine. Olanzapine is approved for the maintenance treatment of schizophrenia and bipolar, for acute and mixed mania, and for bipolar depression (in combination with fluoxetine).

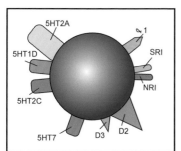

Ziprasidone has actions on 5HT, DA, and norepinephrine (NE) systems. Ziprasidone generally has less weight gain and cardiometabolic risk than some other atypical antipsychotics, as it does not induce weight gain, dyslipidemia, elevation of fasting triglycerides, or insulin resistance. Due to its 5HT2A/D2 blocking capability, it reduces the risk of EPS and elevated prolactin levels. Ziprasidone has been shown to treat both positive and negative symptoms. In cases of acute psychosis, the intramuscular formulation is highly effective. Rapid dose escalation to middle to high doses has been proven most effective. The 5HT1D antagonist actions combined with the 5HT and NE reuptake blocking properties might contribute to its potential antidepressant and anxiolytic properties. Ziprasidone is approved for the treatment of schizophrenia, delaying relapses in schizophrenia, and acute agitation in schizophrenia, as well as acute and mixed mania.

FIGURE 4.14. Properties of some atypical antipsychotics: Part 2.

Properties of Atypical Antipsychotics: Part 3

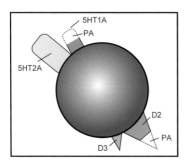

Aripiprazole is the first atypical antipsychotic with D2 partial agonist properties. Its 5HT2A and 5HT1A features may be the reason for its increased tolerability and efficacy. Aripiprazole is effective at treating positive and manic symptoms. Its benefits also lie in its many different formulations (tablets, disintegrating tablets, liquid, and IM formulations). Aripiprazole is usually devoid of sedative side effects, and can even be activating. For some patients aripiprazole is either too close to a full antagonist, or too close to a full agonist. In both cases, dose adjustment and the timing of administration can ameliorate these symptoms. Similarly to ziprasidone, aripiprazole causes little to no weight gain, most likely because it lacks 5HT2C and histamine H1 properties. Additionally, aripiprazole does not seem to induce dyslipidemia, increase fasting triglyceride levels, or increase insulin resistance. Thus aripiprazole has a lower cardiometabolic risk. Aripiprazole is approved for the treatment of schizophrenia (adults and adolescents), maintaining stability in schizophrenia, acute and mixed mania, and bipolar maintenance. It is also approved as an adjunct treatment to antidepressants in major depressive disorder.

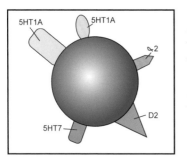

Paliperidone has actions on 5HT, DA, and alpha 2 adrenergic systems. Paliperidone is the active metabolite of risperidone and thus has a similar receptor profile; it is primarily a 5HT2A/D2 antagonist. The oral sustained-release formulation of paliperidone allows it to be taken just once a day. This property will most likely also lead to less extrapyramidal side effects and sedation compared to its parent compound. Paliperidone may improve depression due to its alpha 2 antagonist properties. It might, however, be associated with weight gain, insulin resistance, and diabetes as well as prolactin elevation, similar to risperidone, and therefore requires monitoring of patients. Studies in bipolar disorder are underway but paliperidone is not yet approved for this purpose. Paliperidone is approved for acute and maintenance treatment of schizophrenia.

FIGURE 4.15. Properties of some atypical antipsychotics: Part 3.

Properties of Atypical Antipsychotics: Part 4

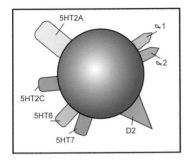

Iloperidone is one of the newer atypical antipsychotics with 5HT2A/D2 antagonistic properties. The doses used in clinical trials have been up to 32 mg/day, with an anticipated dose range of 12-24 mg/day given in divided doses. Similar side effects have been observed throughout the dosage range. Iloperidone exhibits dose-dependent QTc prolongation. Early studies indicate iloperidone's efficacy in schizophrenia may be linked to certain pharmacogenetic markers. This agent has just received FDA approval for the treatment of schizophrenia.

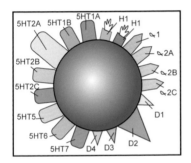

The newly developed atypical antipsychotic **asenapine** has a receptor profile even more complex than that of clozapine. It includes new properties such as actions at 5HT1B/2B receptors and alpha 2A, 2B, and 2C properties. The relevance of actions at all these receptors is not yet known. Asenapine has been developed as a sublingual formulation. Doses of 5 and 10 mg have been tested for mania and schizophrenia. Asenapine shows only mild metabolic risk and no prolactin elevation. This agent is filed with the FDA as of this writing and not yet available for use.

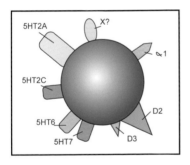

Another atypical antipsychotic with a 5HT2A/D2 antagonism profile is **sertindole**. It has proven beneficial in patients not responding to other treatment; however, patients need to be closely monitored for their cardiac status and drug interactions, as sertindole can increase QTc prolongation. Sertindole is currently not yet available in the United States.

FIGURE 4.16. Properties of some atypical antipsychotics: Part 4.

Cardiometabolic and Sedative Effects

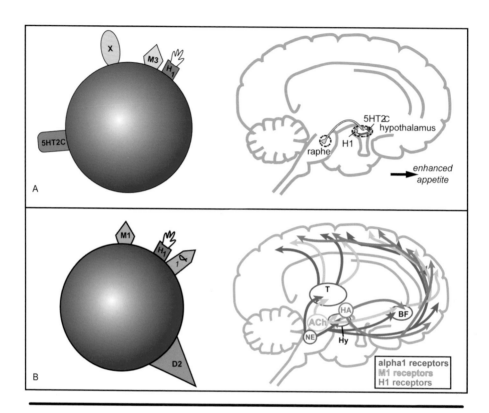

FIGURE 4.17. (A) There are a few receptors that, hypothetically, might increase cardiometabolic risk; these include 5HT2C, M3, and H1 receptors, as well as receptors yet to be identified (signified here as receptor "X"). Specifically, 5HT2C and H1 antagonism is linked to weight gain, and M3 receptor antagonism can alter insulin regulation. Receptor "X" may increase insulin resistance, resulting in elevated fasting plasma triglyceride levels. Some patients might be more prone than others to experience increased cardiometabolic risk on certain atypical antipsychotics. Simultaneous blockade of 5HT2C and H1 receptors can lead to weight gain, which could result from increased appetite stimulation via hypothalamic eating centers. (B) D2, M1, H1, and alpha1 adrenergic receptor antagonism can all lead to sedation. Thus the atypical antipsychotics with those receptor properties will at some level or another alter arousal in patients. Acetylcholine (ACh), histamine (HA), and norepinephrine (NE) are all involved in arousal pathways, thereby connecting neurotransmitter centers with the thalamus (T), hypothalamus (Hy), basal forebrain (BF), and cortex. Thus, it is predictable that atypical antipsychotics with pharmacologic actions that block these receptors could be associated with sedating effects.

Weight Gain and Cardiometabolic
Risk of Mood Stabilizers

Antipsychotic	Weight Gain Risk
Clozapine	+++
Olanzapine	+++
Risperidone*	++
Quetiapine	++
Ziprasidone	+/-
Aripiprazole	+/-

TABLE 4.1. Various mood stabilizers and their risk of weight gain. The information reflects FDA and expert agreement on three tiers of risk.

* Paliperidone (active metabolite of risperidone) carries the same weight gain risk.
+++ high risk
++ intermediate risk
+/- low risk

— ● —

Antipsychotic	Cardiometabolic
Ziprasidone	Low
Aripiprazole	Low
Amisulpride	Possibly low, not well studied
Iloperidone	Possibly low, currently studied
Asenapine	Possibly low, currently studied

TABLE 4.2. Some atypical antipsychotics are "metabolically friendly," in that they are low-risk for both weight gain and cardiometabolic illness.

The Metabolic Highway

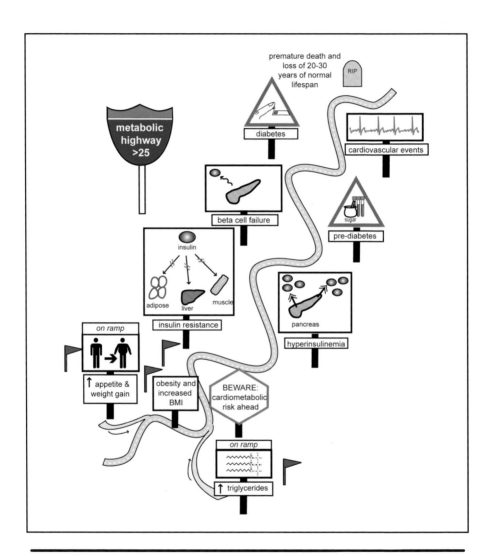

FIGURE 4.18. The metabolic highway depicts different stages that precede cardio-vascular disease and premature death. Increased appetite and weight gain combined with a body mass index greater than 25 is the "entrance ramp" to the highway. The highway will eventually lead down the following path: obesity, insulin resistance, and dyslipidemia with increased fasting triglyceride levels. When hyperinsulinemia leads to pancreatic beta cell failure, prediabetes and then diabetes can ensue. The presence of diabetes increases a patient's risk for cardiovascular events and premature death.

Monitoring and Managing Antipsychotics: Best Practices

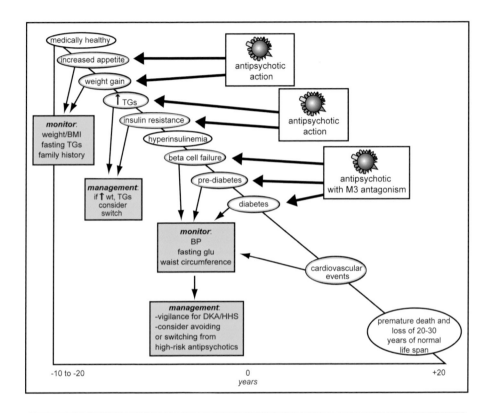

FIGURE 4.19. What are the best practices for monitoring and managing mood stabilizers? Patients who will be dosed with a mood stabilizer should undergo baseline measurements including weight, BMI, fasting triglyceride levels (TGs), and family history of diabetes. Weight, BMI, and fasting triglycerides should be monitored throughout treatment, and if weight or triglyceride levels increase, then the patient should be switched to a different mood stabilizer, have therapeutic lifestyle interventions, or both. When patients have dyslipidemia, are prediabetic or diabetic, or are obese, it is necessary to obtain their fasting glucose levels, blood pressure, and waist circumference measurements just before starting treatment with mood stabilizers and throughout treatment. It may be best in these patients to avoid or switch from mood stabilizers that exhibit a higher risk of cardiometabolic side effects.

BMI: body mass index. DKA: diabetic ketoacidosis. HHS: hyperglycemic state. TGs: triglycerides

The Involvement of a Psychopharmacologist

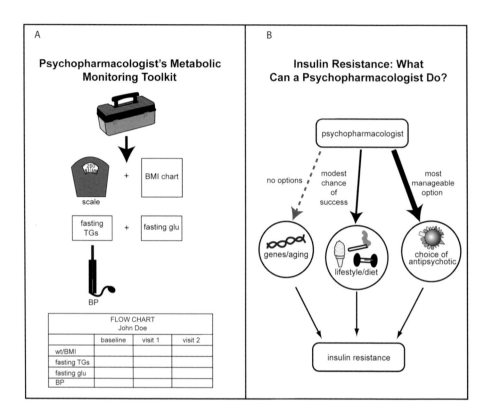

FIGURE 4.20. (A) A simple metabolic toolkit can be used to track the four main parameters: weight/BMI, fasting triglycerides, fasting glucose, and blood pressure. By recording those items at the beginning of treatment and getting regular laboratory tests done for fasting triglycerides and fasting glucose, it is possible to simply monitor a patient and prevent the occurrence of future devastating side effects.

(B) Although a psychopharmacologist can individualize the choice of an atypical antipsychotic, there are various factors that are out of his/her control. These include genetic factors such as age, family history, etc. The psychopharmacologist can also put power into the patients' hands by educating them on lifestyle choices, such as diet, exercise, and smoking. However, the most manageable option for cardiometabolic risk may be which antipsychotic the patient takes.

The Good and the Bad of Sedation

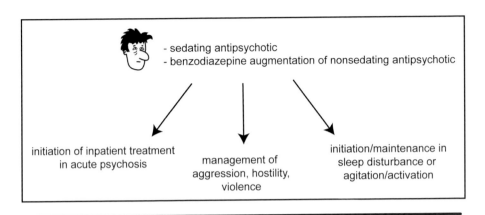

- sedating antipsychotic
- benzodiazepine augmentation of nonsedating antipsychotic

initiation of inpatient treatment in acute psychosis

management of aggression, hostility, violence

initiation/maintenance in sleep disturbance or agitation/activation

FIGURE 4.21. Although it is preferable to avoid long-term sedation, it can be useful initially in the treatment of mania, especially psychotic mania. Short-term sedation can aid in managing acute psychosis, aggression, hostility, violence, sleep disturbances, or agitation/activation. A sedating mood stabilizer or an adjunct benzodiazepine can be used to induce sedation.

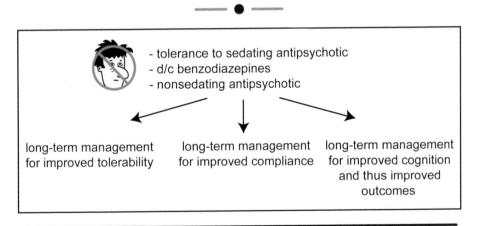

- tolerance to sedating antipsychotic
- d/c benzodiazepines
- nonsedating antipsychotic

long-term management for improved tolerability

long-term management for improved compliance

long-term management for improved cognition and thus improved outcomes

FIGURE 4.22. Long-term sedation, however, is one of the top reasons for discontinuing an antipsychotic for intolerability. Patients whose nonsedating antipsychotic medication was initially augmented with a benzodiazepine may need to discontinue the benzodiazepine. For some patients treated with a sedating antipsychotic, it might be necessary to change their medication. Other patients might become tolerant to the sedating side effects of their medication. Individualized treatment may be necessary in determining the best possible treatment plan for each patient.

How Can Functional Outcome Be Optimized?

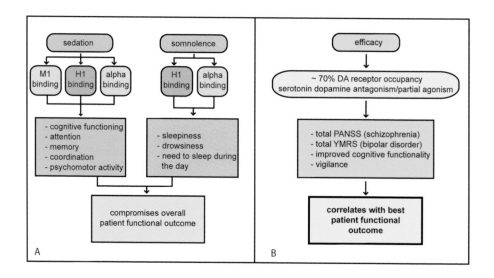

FIGURE 4.23. (A) Blockade of muscarinic M1, histamine H1, and/or alpha1 adrenergic receptors can lead to sedation, which can impact cognitive functioning, attention, memory, and coordination. All of these will result in poor overall functioning for patients with schizophrenia. Somnolence, which can lead to sleepiness and drowsiness, is most likely mediated by blockade of H1 and alpha1 adrenergic receptors. These symptoms can also affect the overall functioning of the patient. (B) An adequate treatment of schizophrenia aims to resolve positive symptoms, as well as affective, cognitive, and negative symptoms. Pharmacologically, this requires approximately 70% blockade of D2 receptors in the nucleus accumbens, in addition to antagonism/partial agonism of D2, 5HT2A, and 5HT1A receptors in other key brain regions. Antagonism of histamine H1, muscarinic M1, or alpha 1 adrenergic receptors is best avoided, as these lead to most of the side effects seen with antipsychotics.

Future Antipsychotics/Mood Stabilizers
on the Horizon, Part 1

Table 4.3. Part 1	
Compounds	**Properties and Notes**
Anticonvulsants	Eslicarbazepine, the active metabolite of oxcarbazepine, has a mechanism related to carbamazepine and is known to be effective in bipolar disorder; JZP-4, a compound related to lamotrigine, is in testing
Glucocorticoid antagonists/ CRF1 antagonists/ V1B antagonists	Blocking stress-inducing increases in glucocorticoids may also block the potentially deleterious effects of glucocorticoids on neurons in bipolar disorder; similarly, blocking corticotrophin releasing factor 1 (CRF1) or vasopressin 1B (V1B) receptors may prevent the adverse consequences of stress on neurons in bipolar disorder
Peptide-linked agents	Neurokinin 1 antagonists have been tested, with unclear benefits; neurokinin 2 antagonist (saredutant) has preliminary evidence of efficacy in unipolar depression, and due to its non-monoaminergic mechanism may also be useful for bipolar depression; neurokinin 3 antagonists are also in testing
Acetylcholine-linked agents	Partial agonists at alpha-7-nicotinic cholinergic receptors may be pro-cognitive agents; varenicline, an alpha-4 beta-2 partial agonist, is approved for smoking cessation and could be beneficial in bipolar disorder
GlyT1 inhibitors	Glycine transporter (GlyT1) inhibitors such as sarcosine block reuptake of glycine, thus increasing its synaptic availability; this could then lead to enhancement of NMDA neurotransmission and reversal of hypofunctioning of NMDA receptors, and theoretically improve cognition

Future Antipsychotics/Mood Stabilizers on the Horizon, Part 2

Table 4.3. Part 2	
Compounds	**Properties and Notes**
New 5HT agents	5HT2A-selective antagonist/inverse agonist, 5HT1A agonist/antagonist and 5HT2C agonist/antagonist are being investigated to improve cognitive effects and reduce side effects; 5HT6 antagonist might be beneficial by increasing brain-derived neurotrophic factor; 5HT7 antagonist could be beneficial for sleep and anxiety
New DA agents	D3 antagonists or partial agonists could potentially be useful to treat negative and cognitive symptoms and to alleviate stimulant abuse; D1 agonists and DA transporter inhibitors may be useful pro-cognitive agents
Glycine agonists	Glycine, d-serine, or its analogue d-cyclosporine bind to the glycine site of the NMDA receptor, and could potentially stimulate the NMDA receptors enough to overcompensate for their hypothetical hypofunction; d-cyclosporine is effective at treating negative and cognitive symptoms
Sigma 1 agonists/ antagonists	Sigma 1 receptors are linked to the psychotomimetic actions of PCP and regulate NMDA receptors; it is not yet known whether an agonist or antagonist would be best in bipolar disorder (the "sigma enigma")
mGluR agents	mGluR2/3 presynaptic receptor agonists could potentially decrease glutamate release; mGluR1 postsynaptic receptor agonists can hypothetically stimulate glutamate receptors and indirectly enhance postsynaptic NMDA-mediated neurotransmission
AMPA-kines	Positive allosteric modulators (PAMs) of this other glutamate receptor subtype, the AMPA receptor, can potentially enhance cognitive functioning

Chapter 5

Bipolar Disorder and Schizophrenia Pharmacy and Switching Strategies

Chapter 5 aims to develop an understanding of the best treatment practices and maintenance methods for optimizing individual patient outcomes in bipolar disorder, and to develop an understanding of the best treatment practices and switching methods for schizophrenia. Determining the best treatment approach for patients with bipolar disorders or schizophrenia can be challenging. Different "pharmacies" that can be useful in the search for an effective treatment plan are presented in this chapter. Practical switching strategies are also presented that will aid in properly changing medications in patients when different treatments are required.

Mood Stabilizers Pharmacy

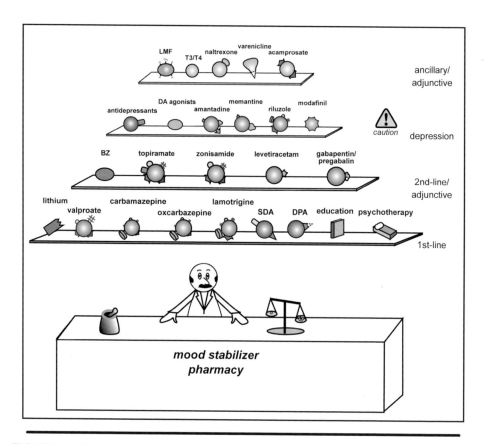

FIGURE 5.1. Current best treatments for bipolar disorder. Although many of these agents have been approved for first-line use as monotherapy, in reality, to treat all symptoms of bipolar disorder, a unique portfolio of two or more treatments is the general rule. Figure 5.5 will elaborate on how to select and combine these treatments.

LMF: l-methylfolate. T3/T4: thyroid hormones. BZ: benzodiazepine. SDA: serotonin-dopamine antagonist. DPA: dopamine partial agonist.

72

Bipolar Mania Pharmacy

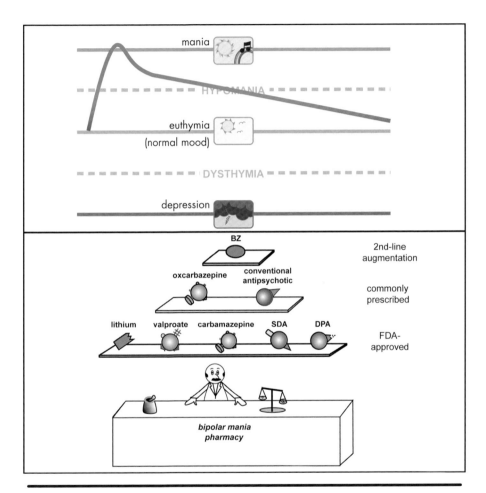

FIGURE 5.2. Current best treatments for acute bipolar mania.

BZ: benzodiazepine. SDA: sertonin-dopamine antagonist. DPA: dopamine partial agonist.

Bipolar Depression Pharmacy

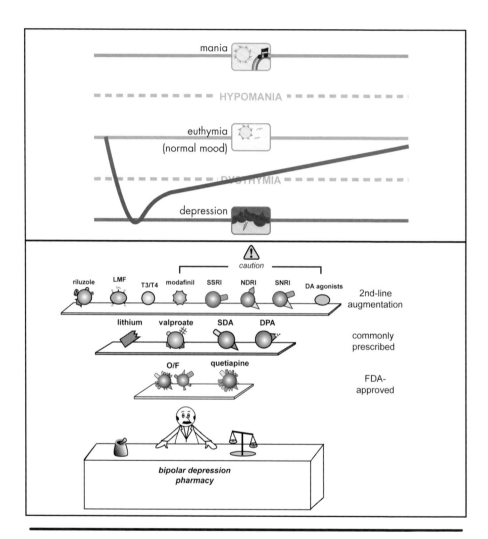

FIGURE 5.3. Current best treatments for bipolar depression.

LMF: l-methylfolate. T3/T4: thyroid hormones. SSRI: selective serotonin reuptake inhibitor. NDRI: norepinephrine and dopamine reuptake inhibitor. DPA: dopamine partial agonist. O/F: olanzapine/fluoxetine combination. SNR: serotonin norepinephrine reuptake inhibitor. SDA: serotonin dopamine antagonist.

Bipolar Maintenance Pharmacy

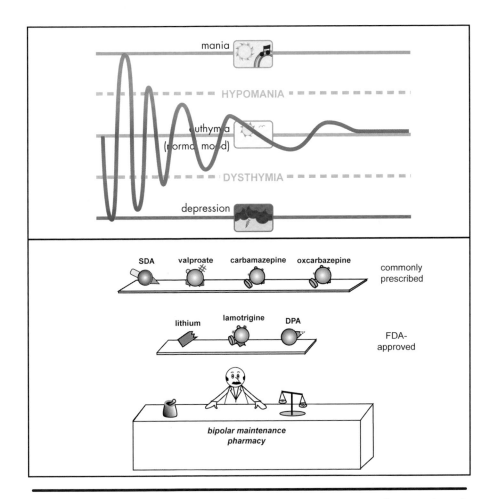

FIGURE 5.4. Current best treatments for long-term maintenance and prevention of manic or depressive episodes.

SDA: serotonin dopamine antagonist. DPA: dopamine partial agonist.

Evidence-based vs. Practice-based Bipolar Combos

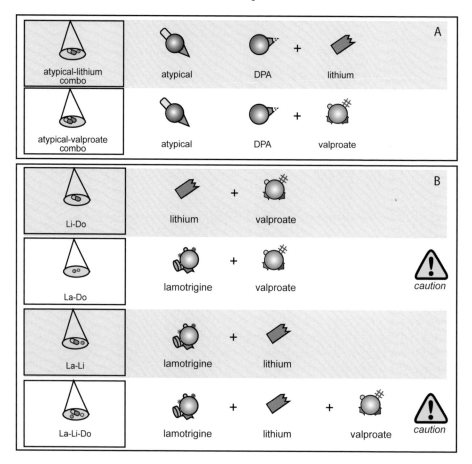

FIGURE 5.5. (A) The best **evidence-based combinations** are those that combine an atypical antipsychotic, especially ones that have been on the market longest, such as olanzapine, risperidone, quetiapine, or aripiprazole, with the addition of lithium or valproate. These four atypicals are FDA-approved as combination therapy with lithium or valproate for manic and mixed episodes. Newer atypicals such as ziprasidone, paliperidone, asenapine, and iloperidone may also be useful in combination with lithium or valproate but are not as well studied. (B) These mood stabilizers have remarkably few controlled studies of their use together. The evidence supporting combinations of these drugs derives from the fact that they have different mechanisms of action and different clinical profiles in the various phases of bipolar disorders. They have been usefully combined in clinical practice according to **practice-based evidence**.

Antidepressants:
Do They Induce Mania?

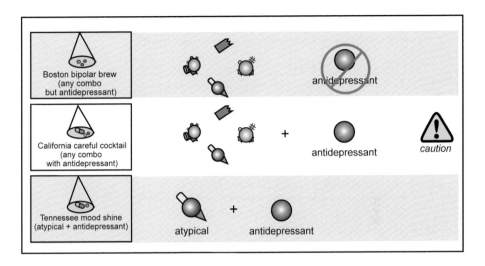

FIGURE 5.6. Recommendations for antidepressant use in patients with known bipolar disorder, who are at risk for bipolar disorder, or who have experienced only antidepressant-induced mania, are still evolving. Currently, use of antidepressants for individuals in these situations must be considered on a case-by-case basis. Most experts agree that antidepressant monotherapy is generally to be avoided in such individuals, and that treatment of depression in bipolar disorder should start with other options such as lamotrigine, lithium, and/or atypical antipsychotics as monotherapies or in combination. Whether one can add an antidepressant to these agents in patients with bipolar depression who do not have robust treatment responses to these first-line agents is a subject of current debate.

Treating Positive and Negative Symptoms of Schizophrenia

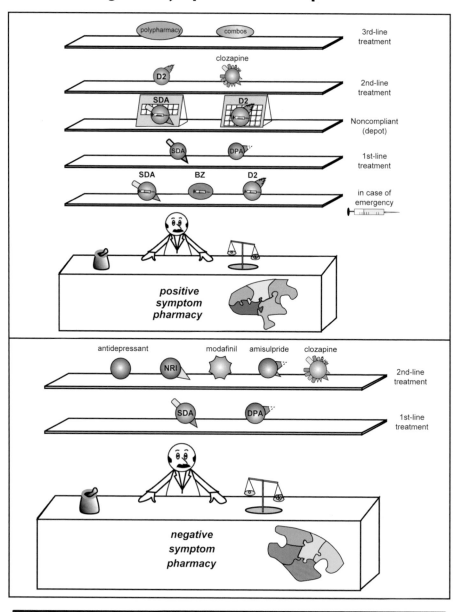

FIGURE 5.7. The best treatment for the positive and negative symptoms of schizophrenia.

Treating Metabolic Issues

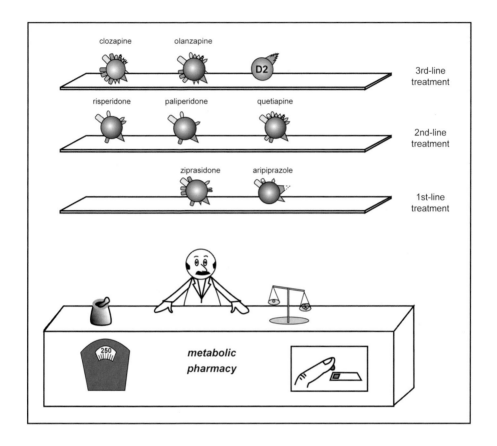

FIGURE 5.8. Aripiprazole and ziprasidone appear to have lower risks for cardiometabolic problems and weight gain, and therefore represent the first-line treatment in the metabolic pharmacy. Risperidone, paliperidone, and quetiapine are second-line treatment options as they carry an intermediate risk of weight gain and the development of cardiometabolic side effects. Olanzapine and clozapine have the highest risk of weight gain and therefore cardiometabolic disease, and should only be used as third-line treatment. Some of the conventional antipsychotics might actually carry less risk of cardiometabolic side effects, but more research is required.

Treating Sedation

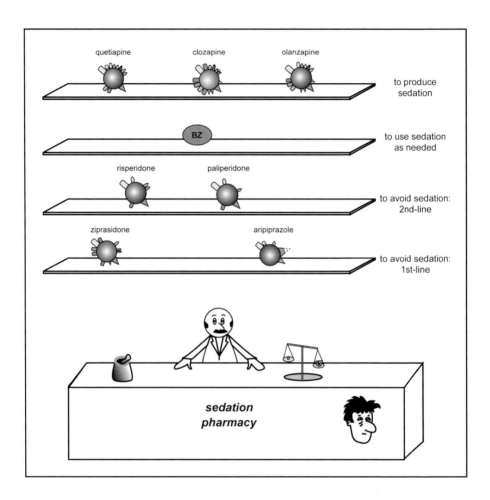

FIGURE 5.9. Ziprasidone and aripiprazole are the antipsychotics with the least tendency to induce sedation. Risperidone and paliperidone have been known to induce sedation in some patients, but not in others. If sedation is wanted, then compounds such as quetiapine, clozapine, or olanzapine should be used. Augmentation with a benzodiazepine can also lead to sedation.

Switching Strategies:
Part 1

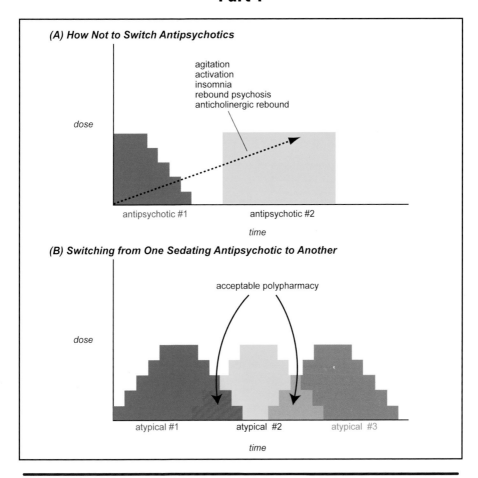

(A) How Not to Switch Antipsychotics

agitation
activation
insomnia
rebound psychosis
anticholinergic rebound

dose

antipsychotic #1   antipsychotic #2

time

(B) Switching from One Sedating Antipsychotic to Another

acceptable polypharmacy

dose

atypical #1   atypical #2   atypical #3

time

FIGURE 5.10. (A) There are strategies for switching antipsychotics and strategies to avoid in order to prevent rebound psychosis, aggravation of side effects, or withdrawal symptoms. Generally, it is preferable to (1) not rush the discontinuation of the first antipsychotic, (2) not allow gaps between two antipsychotic treatments, and (3) not start the second antipsychotic at full dose. (B) Cross-titration is usually advised when switching from one sedating antipsychotic to another. As the first antipsychotic is slowly tapered off, the second antipsychotic is slowly added on. This can be done over a few days or weeks. Even though the patient will be simultaneously taking two medications for a short period of time, this is acceptable as it can decrease side effects and the risk of rebound symptoms, and it can hasten the successful transition to the second drug.

Switching Strategies:
Part 2

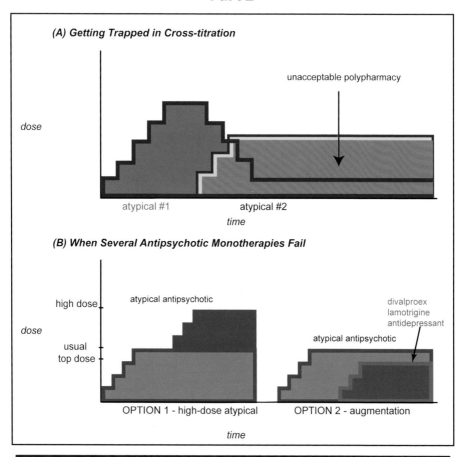

FIGURE 5.11. (A) When initiating cross-titration, it is imperative to not forget to taper the first drug. Patients may improve in the middle of a cross-titration, but this should not be the reason to stop the process. An unfinished cross-titration will lead to polypharmacy where the patient takes two drugs indefinitely. While polypharmacy is sometimes a necessity in hard-to-treat cases, an adequate monotherapy trial of a second drug should be the first option. (B) When a monotherapy with an atypical antipsychotic fails, the psychopharmacologist has few options. Option 1: A high dose of the atypical antipsychotic can be used; however at high doses some side effects might appear that are normally not related to atypical antipsychotics. Option 2: Augmentation with a mood stabilizer such as divalproex or lamotrigine or with an antidepressant could transform a previously ineffective atypical antipsychotic monotherapy into an efficacious drug cocktail.

Switching Strategies:
Part 3

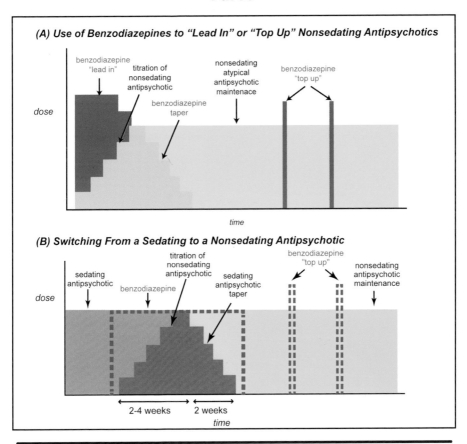

FIGURE 5.12. (A) Benzodiazepines (BZ) can be useful to "lead in" or "top up" a nonsedating antipsychotic. For agitated patients, it may be beneficial to shortly augment with a BZ, and use it as a "lead in" while initiating a nonsedating antipsychotic. Once the nonsedating antipsychotic has been titrated to its full dose, the BZ can be slowly tapered. During the maintenance phase of the antipsychotic it can be helpful to use a BZ as a "top up" when needed by the patient. (B) Switching from a sedating to a nonsedating antipsychotic can be problematic. One method to do so suggests adding a BZ before the nonsedating antipsychotic is titrated to its optimal therapeutic dose, while the sedating antipsychotic is still given at full dose. Once the sedating antipsychotic is slowly tapered and the patient is stable, the BZ can be stopped. "Topping up" can be used sporadically, if agitation or insomnia occur. This switching strategy may be best for patients who are switching due to lack of adequate control of symptoms by their sedating antipsychotic.

Switching Strategies:
Part 4

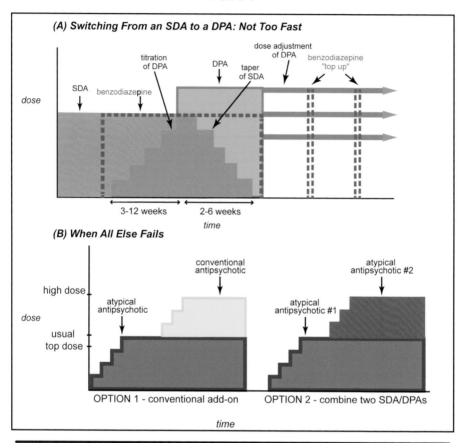

FIGURE 5.13. (A) The emergence of psychosis, agitation, and insomnia can potentially burden the switch from a 5HT2A/D2 antagonist (SDA) to a D2 partial agonist (DPA). The second antipsychotic can be gradually added while keeping the first one at full dose. Adding a benzodiazepine short-term may be beneficial. After a few weeks the SDA can be tapered, and the benzodiazepine stopped. When switching to a DPA, it is important to give the receptors time to adjust their sensitivity, and thus the dose of the DPA may need to be adjusted in order to reach full therapeutic potential. (B) When pushing the dose of an atypical antipsychotic or augmenting it with other drugs still fails, it might be necessary to combine two antipsychotics. A conventional antipsychotic (left), or an atypical antipsychotic such as an SDA or DPA (right) can be added to the first atypical drug. While antipsychotic polypharmacy is frequently practiced, it has not been well studied and should only be used when every other approach has failed.

Psychotherapy in Bipolar Disorder

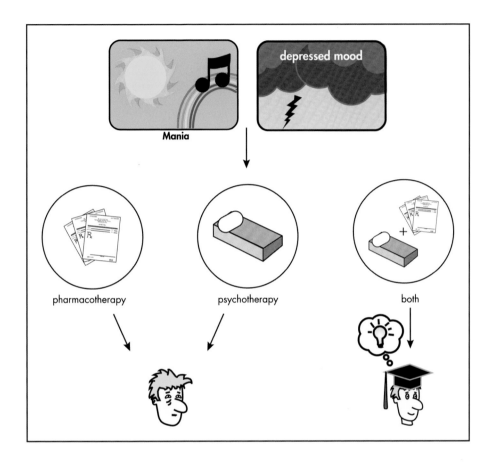

FIGURE 5.14. Psychotherapy adjunct to pharmacotherapy has been shown to improve overall quality-of-life in patients with bipolar disorder. Behavioral and educational therapies help improve factors such as total functioning, relationship functioning, life satisfaction, compliance with medication, and personal coping mechanisms. Psychotherapy can provide a necessary regular forum for patients to express and work through the progression of their illness and the coping mechanisms they use to overcome their limitations.

Summary

- Bipolar disorder can be difficult to spot as symptoms with which patients present often appear quite similar to unipolar depression, anxiety, or other psychiatric illnesses.

- The underlying pathophysiology of schizophrenia remains to be fully elucidated; but dopamine, glutamate, and serotonin are three of the most important neurotransmitter systems involved in schizophrenia and in the mechanisms of action of conventional and atypical antipsychotics.

- In order to optimize treatment in both disorders, it is necessary to understand the neurobiological basis of symptoms and the pharmacologic mechanisms of action involved in correcting that abnormal neurobiology.

- Each mood-stabilizer and antipsychotic has a unique receptor profile, important in the alleviation of symptoms and induction of side effects.

- Successfully targeting the right neural circuits in individual cases as well as selecting and combining treatments for optimal outcomes is psychopharmacological art.

- Throughout treatment, it is critical to track and monitor patients to determine the effectiveness of the patient's treatment plan and to evaluate the progression of illness.

- Combining psychotherapy with pharmacotherapy may synergistically work to improve quality-of-life, which in addition to treating a disorder is the ultimate goal of any treatment plan.

References

Agid O, Mamo D, Ginovart N, Vitcu I, Wilson AA, Zipursky RB et al. Neuropsychopharmacology 2007;32:1209–15.

Alphs LD, Summerfelt A, Lann H, Muller RJ. Psychopharmacol Bull1989;25(2):159–63.

Altshuler LL, Bookheimer SY, Townsend J, Proenza MA, Eisenberger N, Sabb F et al. Biol Psychiatry 2005;58:763–9.

Angst J. British Journal of Psychiatry 2007;190:189–91.

Artaloytia JF, Arango C, Lahti A, Sanz J, Pascual A, Cubero P et al. Am J Psychiatry 2006;163(3):48–93.

Atmaca M, Kuloglu M, Tezcan E, Ustundag B. J Clin Psychiatry 2003;64(5):598–604.

Baumer FM, Howe M, Gallelli K, Simeonova DI, Hallmayer J, Chang KD. Biol Psychiatry 2006;60:1005–12.

Bardin L, Kleven MS, Barret-Grevoz C, Depoortere R, Newman-Tancredi A. Neuropsychopharmacology 2006;31:1869–79.

Bennett S, Gronier B. Eur J Pharmacol 2005;527:52–9.

Biederman J, Mick E, Hammerness P, Harpold T, Aleardi M, Dougherty M et al. Biol Psychiatry 2005;58:589–94.

Bota RG, Sagduyu K, Munro JS. CNS Spectr 2005;10(12):937–42.

Calabrese JR, Shelton MD, Rapport DJ, Youngstrom EA, Jackson K, Bilali S et al. Am J Psychiatry 2005;162:2152–61.

Chiu CC, Chen KP, Liu HC, Lu ML. J Clin Psychopharmacol 2006;26(5):504–7.

Cipriani A, Pretty H, Hawton K, Geddes JR. Am J Psychiatry 2005;162:1805–19.

Citrome L, Jaffe A, Levine J, Martello D. Psychiatr Serv 2006;57(8)1132–9.

Cousins DA, Young AH. Intl J Neuropsychopharmacology 2007;10:411–31.

Coyle JT, Tsai G, Goff D. Ann N Y Acad Sci 2003;1003:318–27.

Coyle JT. Cell Mol Neurobiol 2006;26(4–6):365–84.

De Bartolomeis A, Fiore G, Iasevoli F. Curr Pharm Design 2005;11:3561–94.

Delbello MP, Adler CM, Whitsel RM, Stanford KE, Strakowski SM. J Clin Psychiatry 2007;68(5):789–95.

Delbello MP, Hanseman D, Adler CM, Fleck DE, Strakowski SM. Am J Psychiatry 2007;164:582–90.

Delbello MP, Kowatch RA, Adler CM, Stanford KE, Welge JA, Barzman DH et al. J Am Acad Child Adolesc Psychiatry 2006;45(3):305–13.

DiForti M, Lappin JM, Murray RM. Eur Neuropsychopharmacol 2007;17:S101–7.

Du J, Suzuki K, Wei Y, Wang Y, Blumenthal R, Chen Z et al. Neuropsychopharmacology 2007;32:793–802.

Essock SM, Covell NH, Davis SM, Stroup TS, Rosenheck RA, Lieberman JA. Am J Psychiatry 2006;163(12):2090–5.

Glenthoj BY, Mackeprang T, Svarer C, Rasmussen H, Pinborg LH, Friberg L et al. Biol Psychiatry 2006;60:621–9.

Houseknecht KL, Robertson AS, Zavadoski W, Gibbs EM, Johnson DE, Rollema H. Neuro psychopharmacology 2007;32:289–97.

Javitt DC. Curr Opin Psychiatry 2006;19:151–7.

Jindal RD, Keshavan S. J Clin Psychopharmacol 2006;26(5):449–50.

Jones PB, Barnes TRE, Davies L, Dunn G, Lloyd H, Hayhurst KP et al. Arch Gen Psychiatry 2006;63:1079–87.

Kahn RS, Schulz SC, Palazov VD, Reyes EB, Brecher M, Svensson O et al. J Clin Psychiatry 2007;68(6):832–42.

Kalkman HO, Feuerbach D, Lotscher E, Schoeffter P. Life Sci 2003;73:1151–9.

Keefe RS, Bilder RM, Davis SM, Harvey PD, Palmer BW, Gold JM et al. Arch Gen Psychiatry 2007;64:633–47.

Keefe RS, Seidman LJ, Christensen BK, Harner RM, Sharma T, Sitskoorn MM et al. Biol Psychiatry 2006;59:97–105.

Kern RS, Green MF, Cornblatt BA, Owen JR, McQuade RD, Carson WH et al. Psychopharmacology 2006;187:312–20.

Kessing LV, Søndergård L, Kvist K, Andersen PK. Arch Gen Psychiatry 2005;62:860–6.

Kessler RM, Ansari MS, Riccardi P, Li R, Jayathilake K, Dawant B et al. Neuropsychopharmacology 2006;31:1991–2001.

Lambert BL, Cunningham FE, Miller DR, Dalack GW, Hur K. Am J Epidemiol 2006;164:672–81.

Lawler CP, Prioleau C, Lewis MM, Mak C, Jiang D, Schetz JA et al. Neuropsychopharmacology 1999;20(6):612–27.

Leucht S, Busch R, Math D, Kissling W, Kane JM. J Clin Psychiatry 2007;68(3):352–60.

Lieberman JA, Stroup TS, McEvoy JP, Swartz MS, Rosenheck RA, Perkins DO et al. N Engl J Med 2005;353(12):1209–23.

References (cont.)

Lindenmayer JP, Khan A, Iskander A, Abad MT, Parker B. J Clin Psychiatry 2007;68(3):368–79.

Lipkovich I, Citrome L, Perlis R, Deberdt W, Jouston JP, Ahl J et al. J Clin Psychopharmocol 2006;26(3):316–20.

Lynch G, Gall CM. Trends Neurosci 2006;29:10.

McCreary AD, Glennon JC, Ashby Jr R, Meltzer HY, Li Z, Reinders JH et al. Neuropsychopharmacology 2007;32:78–94.

McGlashan TH, Zipursky RB, Perkins D, Addington J, Miller T, Woods SW et al. Am J Psychiatry 2006;163:790–9.

Meyer JM, Stahl SM. Acta Psychiatr Scand. 2009;119(1):4–14.

Millan MJ. Psychopharmacology 2005;179:30–53.

Miklowitz DJ, Otto MW, Frank E, Reilly-Harrington NA, Kogan JN, Sachs GS et al. Am J Psychiatry 2007;164(9):1340–7.

Mizrahi R, Rusjan P, Agid O, Graff A, Mamo DC, Zipursky RB et al. Am J Psychiatry 2007;164:630–7.

Natesan S, Reckless GE, Nobrega JN, Fletcher PJ, Kapur S. Neuropsychopharmacology 2006;31:1854–63.

Newman-Tancredi A, Assie MB, Leduc N, Ormiere AM, Danty N, Cosi C. Int J Neuropsychopharmacol 2005;8:341–56.

Nierenberg AA, Ostacher MJ, Borrelli DJ, Iosifescu DV, Perlis RH, Desrosiers A et al. J Clin Psychiatry 2006;67(Suppl 11):3–7.

Nierenberg AA, Ostacher MJ, Calabrese JR, Ketter TA, Marangell LB, Miklowitz DJ et al. Am J Psychiatry 2006;163:210–6.

Oquendo MA, Currier D, Mann JJ. Acta Psychiatr Scand 2006;114:151–8.

Olfson M, Marcus SC, Corey-Lisle P, Tuomari AV, Hines P, L'Italien GJ. Am J Psychiatry 2006;163:1821–5.

Perlis RH, Ostacher MJ, Patel JK, Marangell LB, Zhang H, Wisniewski SR et al. Am J Psychiatry 2006;163:217–24.

Pierre JM, Peloian JH, Wirshing DA,Wirshing WC, Marder SR. J Clin Psychiatry 2007;68(5):705–10.

Reist C, Mintz J, Albers LJ, Jamas MM, Szabo S, Ozdemir V. J Clin Psychopharmacol 2007;27:46–51.

Remington G, Mamo D, Labelle A, Reiss J, Shammi C, Mannaert E et al. Am J Psychiatry 2006;163(3):396–401.

Reynolds GP, Yao Z, Zhang XB, Sun J, Zhang ZJ. Eur Neuropsychopharmacol 2004;15:143–51.

Sarter M. Trends Pharmacol Sci 2006;27:11.

Sepehry AA, Potvin S, Elie R, Stip E. J Clin Psychiatry 2007;68(4):604–10.

Spurling RD, Lamberti JS, Olsen D, Tu X, Tang W. J Clin Psychiatry 2007;68(3):406–9.

Stahl SM. J Clin Psychiatry 2004;65(11):1445–6.

Stahl SM. Stahl's Essential Psychopharmacology, 3rd Edition, Cambridge University Press, N.Y., 2008.

Stahl SM. Stahl's Essential Psychopharmacology: Prescriber's Guide, 3rd Edition, Cambridge University Press, N.Y., 2009.

Stahl SM, Mignon L, Meyer JM. Acta Psychiatr Scand. 2009;119(3):171–9.

Stroup TS, Lieberman JA, McEvoy JP, Swartz MS, Davis SM, Capuano GA et al. Am J Psychiatry 2007;164:415–27.

Takahashi H, Higuchi M, Suhara T. Biol Psychiatry 2006;59:919–28.

Talkowski ME, Mansour H, Chowdari KV, Wood J, Butler A, Varma PG et al. Biol Psychiatry 2006;60:570–7.

Tenback DE, van Harten PN, Sloof CJ, van Os J. Am J Psychiatry 2006;163:1438–40.

Thase ME, Macfadden W, Weisler RH, Chang W, Paulsson B, Khan A et al. J Clin Psychopharmacol 2006;26:600–9.

Tran-Johnson TK, Sack DA, Marcus RN, Auby P, McQuade RD, Oren DA. J Clin Psychiatry 2007;68(1):111–9.

Wagner KD, Kowatch RA, Emslie GJ, Findling RL, Wilens TE, McCague K et al. Am J Psychiatry 2006;163:1179–86.

Weisler RH, Cutler AJ, Ballenger JC, Post RM, Ketter TA. CNS Spectrums 2006;11(10):788–99.

Weissman MM. Am J Psychiatry 2007;164(5)693–6.

West AR, Floresco SB, Charara A, Rosenkranz JA, Grace AA. Ann NY Acad Sci 2003;1003:53-74.

Yatham LN, Goldstein JM, Vieta E, Bowden CL, Grunze H, Post RM et al. J Clin Psychiatry 2005;66(Suppl 5):40–8.

Zhang M, Ballard ME, Kohlhaas KL, Browmna KE, Jongen-Relo AL, Unger LV et al. Neuropsychopharmacology 2006;31:1382–92.

CME Posttest

To receive your certificate of CME credit or participation, please complete the posttest (you must score at least 70% to receive credit) and activity evaluation answer sheet found on the last page and return it by mail or fax it to 760-931-8713. Once received, your posttest will be graded and, along with your certificate (if a score of 70% or more was attained), returned to you by mail. Alternatively, you may complete these items online and immediately print your certificate at **www.neiglobal.com/cme**. There is no fee for CME credits for this activity. **Please circle the correct answer on the answer sheet provided.**

1. A patient presents with delusions and hallucinations. These positive symptoms are hypothesized to result from:
   A. Mesolimbic dopamine hypoactivity
   B. Mesolimbic dopamine hyperactivity
   C. Mesocortical dopamine hypoactivity
   D. Mesocortical dopamine hyperactivity

2. In the "bipolar storm" excessive _____ release from neuron A to neuron B results in unstable and excessive neurotransmission.
   A. Dopamine
   B. GABA
   C. Glutamate
   D. Norepinephrine

3. If glutamate and GABA neurotransmission needs to be modulated, which medication would be able to do so?
   A. Lamotrigine
   B. Levetiracetam
   C. Oxcarbazepine
   D. Valproate

4. Which symptoms of bipolar disorder are due to inefficient information processing in the dorsolateral prefrontal cortex (DLPFC)?
   A. Distractibility/trouble concentrating and executive dysfunction
   B. Executive dysfunction and decreased need for sleep
   C. Decreased need for sleep and depressed mood
   D. Depressed mood and distractibility/trouble concentrating

5. Oxcarbazepine has been used off label because it has a similar mechanism of action as carbamazepine but exhibits a better tolerability profile. However, licarbazepine, not oxcarbazepine, is thought to be responsible for its therapeutic actions. What is the relationship between oxcarbazepine and licarbazepine?
   A. Oxcarbazepine is the racemic; licarbazepine is the enantiomer
   B. Oxcarbazepine is the prodrug; licarbazepine is the active molecule
   C. Oxcarbazepine is the parent drug; licarbazepine is the metabolite

CME Posttest (cont.)

6. The release of dopamine can be increased by:
   A. Stimulation of 5HT1A and 5HT2A receptors
   B. Stimulation of 5HT1A receptors or blockade of 5HT2A receptors
   C. Blockade of 5HT1A receptors or stimulation of 5HT2A receptors
   D. Blockade of 5HT1A and 5HT2A receptors

7. A patient presents with a depressed mood and feelings of guilt and worthlessness. Inefficient information processing of monoamines in which brain areas could hypothetically best explain these symptoms?
   A. Striatum and orbitofrontal cortex
   B. Amygdala and ventromedial prefrontal cortex
   C. Nucleus accumbens and dorsolateral prefrontal cortex
   D. Basal forebrain and anterior cingulate cortex

8. A patient has problems with feeling tired and sleepy all the time. Drugs with which receptors should be taken with caution, if sedation is to be prevented?
   A. D3 and 5HT2A
   B. D1 and 5HT2C
   C. H1 and alpha 1
   D. H3 and alpha 2

9. An obese patient with bipolar disorder needs to be augmented with an atypical antipsychotic. It is best to choose an atypical antipsychotic with the least affinity at receptors that can hypothetically lead to cardiometabolic risk. These include:
   A. D2 and 5HT2A
   B. H1 and 5HT2C
   C. M2 and alpha 1
   D. 5HT3 and alpha 2

10. A recommended strategy for using a benzodiazepine in a patient with schizophrenia is when:
   A. Switching between sedating antipsychotics
   B. One is trapped in cross-titration of antipsychotics
   C. Switching from a sedating to a nonsedating antipsychotic
   D. Everything else fails

From Neurobiology to Treatment: Bipolar Disorder and Schizophrenia Unraveled
Posttest and Activity Evaluation Answer Sheet

Please complete the posttest and activity evaluation answer sheet on this page and return by mail or fax. Alternatively, you may complete these items online and immediately print your certificate at www.neiglobal.com/cme. (Please circle the correct answer)

Posttest Answer Sheet (score of 70% or higher required for CME credit)

1.	A B C D	6.	A B C D
2.	A B C D	7.	A B C D
3.	A B C D	8.	A B C D
4.	A B C D	9.	A B C D
5.	A B C	10.	A B C D

Activity Evaluation: Please rate the following, using a scale of:

1-poor   2-below average   3-average   4-above average   5-excellent

1. The overall quality of the <u>content</u> was…   1 2 3 4 5

2. The overall quality of this <u>activity</u> was…   1 2 3 4 5

3. The relevance of the content to my professional needs was…   1 2 3 4 5

4. The level at which the learning objective was met of teaching me to   1 2 3 4 5
   describe the hypothetical neurobiology of bipolar disorders and the
   complex pharmacology of mood stabilizers used to treat them…

5. The level at which the learning objective was met of teaching me to   1 2 3 4 5
   recognize how different drugs affect the various disease states of bipolar
   disorders and identify mechanisms as well as therapeutic benefits and
   nuances of drugs commonly prescribed for bipolar disorder…

6. The level at which the learning objective was met of teaching me to   1 2 3 4 5
   develop an understanding of the best treatment practices and maintenance
   methods for optimizing individual patient outcome in bipolar disorder…

7. The level at which the learning objective was met of teaching me to   1 2 3 4 5
   describe the hypothetical neurobiology of schizophrenia and understand
   the complex pharmacology of antipsychotics…

8. The level at which the learning objective was met of teaching me to   1 2 3 4 5
   recognize how different drug properties affect the various symptoms of
   schizophrenia and that side effects are linked to the drug's receptor profile…

9. The level at which the learning objective was met of teaching me to develop   1 2 3 4 5
   an understanding of the best treatment practices and switching methods
   in schizophrenia…

10. The level at which this activity was objective, scientifically balanced,   1 2 3 4 5
    and free of commercial bias was…

From Neurobiology to Treatment: Bipolar Disorder and Schizophrenia Unraveled
Posttest and Activity Evaluation Answer Sheet (cont.)

11. Based on my experience and knowledge, the level of this activity was…

     Too Basic   Basic   Appropriate   Complex   Too Complex

12. My confidence level in treating this topic has _____ as a result of participation in this activity.
    A. Increased
    B. Stayed the same
    C. Decreased

13. Based on the information presented in this activity, I will…
    A. Change my practice
    B. Seek additional information on this topic
    C. Do nothing as current practice reflects activity's recommendations
    D. Do nothing as the content was not convincing

14. What barriers might keep you from implementing changes in your practice you'd like to make as a result of participating in this activity?

15. The following additional information about this topic would help me in my practice:

16. How could this activity have been improved?

17. Number of credits I am claiming, commensurate with the extent of my participation in the activity (maximum of 3.0): _____

Name: _____ Credentials: _____

Address: _____

City, State, Zip: _____

Email: _____ Phone: _____

Mail or fax **both sides** of this form to:

Mail: CME Department   Fax: 760-931-8713
         Neuroscience Education Institute   Attn: CME Department
         1930 Palomar Point Way, Suite 101
         Carlsbad, CA 92008